MULTIPLE MYELOMA

DIET COOKBOOK

FOR BEGINNERS

Nourishing Recipes with Expert Guidance for Optimal Health and Healing

Kingsley Klopp

To show our appreciation for your purchase, we're delighted to offer you these special bonuses as a heartfelt thank you

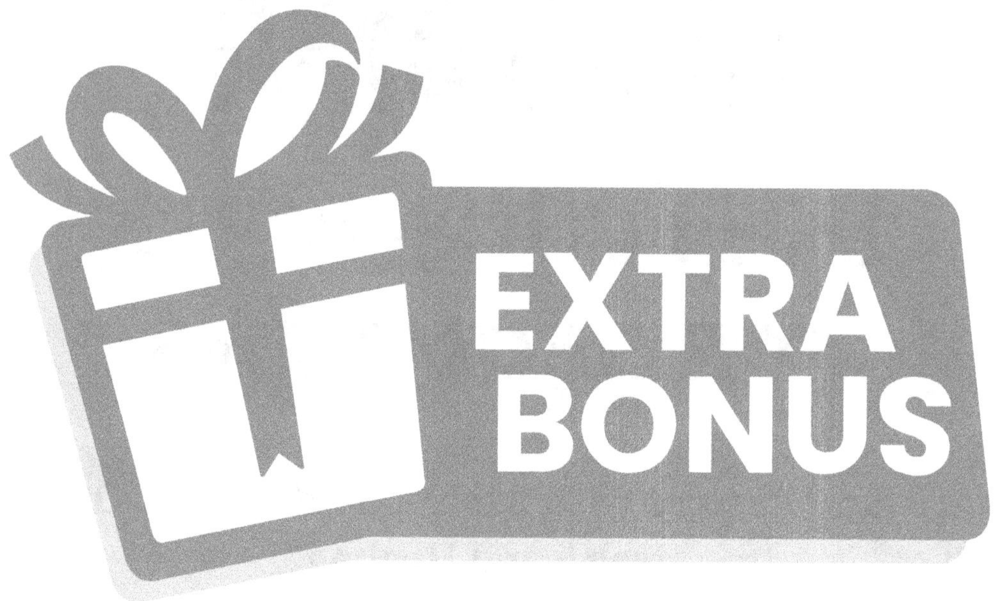

1. A Food Tracker Journal
2. Downloadable E-BOOK featuring full-color images of finished recipes

Table of Content

Introduction..7

Chapter 1: Understanding Multiple Myeloma
- What is Multiple Myeloma?...9
- Symptoms and Diagnosis...11
- Treatment Options..13

Chapter 2: The Role of Nutrition in Multiple Myeloma
- How Diet Affects Multiple Myeloma...15
- Foods to Include and Avoid...17

Breakfast Recipes
Blueberry Almond Smoothie...19
Berry Beet Smoothie...20
Oatmeal with Walnuts and Berries..20
Creamy Buckwheat Porridge...21
Millet Porridge with Honey and Nuts...21
Soft Scrambled Eggs...22
Egg White Omelette with Spinach...23
Silken Tofu Scramble..24
Poached Eggs over Asparagus...25
Greek Yogurt with Mixed Berries..25
Kefir with Honey and Almonds..26
Yogurt Parfait with Muesli...26
Avocado Toast with Sesame Seeds..27
Hummus and Cucumber Sandwich..27
Banana Oat Pancakes...28
Fruit Salad with Mint...29
Melon and Prosciutto Plate..29
Coconut Yogurt and Mango..30
Almond Flour Waffles...31
Cottage Cheese Pancakes..32
Buckwheat Pancakes with Honey..33

Steamed Vegetable Medley..34
Sautéed Mushrooms...35
Whole Grain Waffles...36

Fish Recipes

Baked Salmon with Dill and Lemon..37
Grilled Tuna Steaks with Olive Tapenade..38
Poached Cod in Tomato Broth...39
Herb-Crusted Tilapia...40
Shrimp and Quinoa Salad..41
Mackerel Pate..42
Trout Almondine...43
Haddock in Parchment with Vegetables...44
Salmon Berry Salad...45
Sole Meuniere..46
Asian-Style Steamed Snapper..47
Peppered Mackerel with Horseradish Cream..48
Baked Trout with Herb Butter...49
Lemon Garlic Tilapia..50
Moroccan Spiced Salmon..51
Shrimp Gazpacho..52
Sea Bass with Fennel and Orange..53
Cod with Parsley Pesto..54
Salmon Quiche with Dill...55
Prawn Stir-Fry with Bell Peppers...56
Tilapia with Mango Salsa..57
Flounder Piccata...58
Halibut with Tomato Caper Sauce..59
Miso-Glazed Cod...60
Lemon Baked Perch...61
Ginger Soy Marinated Tuna...62
Pistachio-Crusted Salmon...63
Anchovy Pasta with Garlic and Olive Oil..64

Poultry Recipes

Lemon Herb Roasted Chicken..65
Turkey and Spinach Meatballs...66
Chicken Ginger Soup..67
Baked Chicken with Prunes and Olives..68
Grilled Turkey Burgers...69
Chicken Salad with Avocado..70
Turkey Chili...71

Poached Chicken and Vegetable Salad...72
Chicken Cacciatore...73
Stuffed Turkey Breast..74
Roast Turkey with Citrus Glaze...75
Chicken Pho..76
Moroccan Turkey Stew..77
Turkey and Quinoa Stuffed Peppers...78
Turkey Piccata...79
Herb Roasted Chicken Thighs...80
Chicken and Broccoli Stir-Fry...81
Garlic Lemon Turkey Cutlets...82
Chicken Curry with Coconut Milk...83
Smoked Turkey Breast..84
Turkey Meatloaf with Spinach...85
Balsamic Glazed Turkey Drumsticks...86
Turkey Bolognese over Zucchini Noodles...87
Chicken Pot Pie with Phyllo Crust..88
Roasted Chicken with Squash and Cranberries....................................89

Vegetables

Roasted Brussels Sprouts with Balsamic Glaze.....................................90
Carrot Ginger Soup...91
Spiced Sweet Potato Wedges..92
Beet and Goat Cheese Salad...93
Cauliflower Steak with Herb Sauce...94
Butternut Squash Risotto...95
Sauteed Green Beans with Garlic..96
Eggplant Parmesan Stacks...97
Spaghetti Squash with Tomato Sauce..98
Creamed Spinach..99
Broccoli and Cashew Stir-Fry..100
Kale Salad with Avocado and Pomegranate...101
Mushroom and Barley Pilaf..102
Garlic Roasted Potatoes...103
Bok Choy with Ginger Soy Sauce...104
Kabocha Squash Curry...105

Soup & Stew Recipes

Lentil and Spinach Soup...106
Beef and Barley Soup..107
Vegetable Beef Stew..108
Split Pea Soup with Ham..109

Italian White Bean and Kale Soup...110
Turkey and Wild Rice Soup...111
Mushroom and Thyme Soup...112
Beetroot and Cabbage Borscht..113
Thai Coconut Chicken Soup (Tom Kha Gai)...114
Fisherman's Soup with Tomato and Saffron..115
Sweet Potato and Black Bean Chili...116
Pea and Ham Hock Soup...117
Italian Sausage and Tortellini Soup..118
Winter Vegetable Stew..119
Spiced Chickpea Stew...120
Russian Mushroom and Potato Soup..121

10-WEEK MEAL PLAN..122

Important Note

 We understand that navigating a new diet while managing multiple myeloma can be challenging, and we are here to provide you with delicious and nutritious options to help you along the way.

However, it is important to remember that individual dietary needs and responses can vary significantly. What works well for one person may not be suitable for another. Therefore, we encourage you to listen to your body and adjust the recipes to fit your personal needs and preferences. Your health and comfort are our top priorities.

We strongly recommend consulting with your healthcare provider or a registered dietitian before making any significant changes to your diet. They can offer personalized advice tailored to your specific condition and overall health status, ensuring that you make informed decisions that best support your journey with multiple myeloma.

Additionally, please keep in mind that the nutritional information provided in this cookbook is approximate. Variations in ingredients, brands, and preparation methods can lead to differences in the final nutritional content of your meals. While we strive to offer accurate and helpful data, slight deviations are always possible.

Furthermore, If our cookbook has brought joy to your kitchen and table, we'd be thrilled to hear about your experiences in an Amazon review. On the flip side, if you stumble upon any hiccups while exploring our recipes, don't hesitate to get in touch at **kloppkingsley@gmail.com**. We're here to support your cooking journey every step of the

Our goal is to empower you with the knowledge and tools to create meals that not only nourish your body but also bring joy to your dining experience. We hope this cookbook serves as a valuable resource, inspiring you to explore new flavors and discover dishes that make you feel your best.

Thank you for allowing us to be a part of your wellness journey. Wishing you good health and happy cooking!

Introduction

Welcome to the **Multiple Myeloma Diet Cookbook for Beginners.** If you or someone you care about is grappling with multiple myeloma, you're likely feeling a mix of emotions—fear, hope, confusion, determination. This book is here to be a beacon of support, guiding you through the maze of dietary choices with compassion and clarity. Living with multiple myeloma can feel overwhelming, but the food you eat can be a powerful ally in your battle. Imagine each meal as a weapon in your arsenal, each nutrient a piece of armor bolstering your body's defenses. Food isn't just sustenance; it's medicine, capable of fortifying you from within. This cookbook is crafted to transform your approach to eating, turning every bite into a step towards strength and resilience. The journey with multiple myeloma is deeply personal and often daunting. The medical treatments and regimens you undergo are critical, but so too is what you put on your plate. Proper nutrition can help manage symptoms, boost your immune system, and improve your overall quality of life. The recipes in this book are not just designed to nourish your body, but also to bring you joy and comfort, essential components in any healing process.

Why focus on a cookbook? Because food is a universal comfort, a daily ritual that can be transformed into a healing practice. This book is filled with recipes tailored to support the unique nutritional needs of multiple myeloma patients. They are simple, delicious, and crafted to provide the vitamins, minerals, and other nutrients that your body needs to stay strong and fight back. This cookbook is for everyone touched by multiple myeloma—patients, caregivers, family, and friends. It's a resource to help you make informed, healthful choices in the kitchen, offering meals that are both therapeutic and enjoyable. Whether you're new to this diagnosis or have been managing it for years, you'll find valuable guidance and fresh ideas to invigorate your diet. The recipes here are designed to be more than just food. They are part of a holistic approach to living with multiple myeloma, integrating the latest nutritional science with the comforting familiarity of home-cooked meals. From energizing breakfasts that set a positive tone for the day, to soothing dinners that provide comfort and nourishment, each recipe is a step towards better health and a brighter outlook. Food has an extraordinary ability to connect us to moments of joy, comfort, and even healing. Think of your favorite dish, the one that warms your heart and soul. This cookbook aims to bring that sense of warmth and security to your daily meals, turning each bite into a testament to your resilience and courage.

Navigating multiple myeloma requires strength, and part of that strength comes from what you eat. This book will help you understand the importance of nutrition in managing your condition, offering practical advice on what to eat and what to avoid. It's filled with tips for building a balanced diet, incorporating superfoods, staying hydrated, and managing treatment side effects through thoughtful dietary choices.

By opening this book, you are taking an active role in your health. You are choosing to fight with every meal, to nourish your body and spirit with foods that support your journey. This isn't just a cookbook—it's a companion, a guide, a source of inspiration. It's a testament to the power of food and the strength within you. Let's embark on this journey together. Let's explore the healing power of food, one recipe at a time. Here's to nourishment, to strength, and to hope. Welcome to the **Multiple Myeloma Diet Cookbook for Beginners.** Together, we can make each meal a step toward healing.

Chapter 1: Understanding Multiple Myeloma

What is Multiple Myeloma?

Multiple Myeloma is a complex and challenging form of cancer that originates in the plasma cells of the bone marrow. Plasma cells, a type of white blood cell, play a crucial role in our immune system by producing antibodies that help fight off infections. In multiple myeloma, these plasma cells become abnormal, multiplying uncontrollably and accumulating in the bone marrow. This accumulation disrupts the production of normal blood cells, leading to a cascade of health issues that can profoundly impact a patient's life.

The origins of multiple myeloma are shrouded in the intricate dance of genetics and environmental factors. Researchers believe that a series of genetic mutations trigger the transformation of healthy plasma cells into malignant ones. These mutations are often linked to changes in specific chromosomes and genes, such as the immunoglobulin heavy chain gene, which is critical for antibody production. The precise cause of these genetic changes remains a mystery, but it is clear that they set the stage for the development of this formidable disease. As multiple myeloma progresses, it infiltrates the bone marrow, the soft, spongy tissue inside our bones where blood cells are produced. This invasion leads to the formation of tumors called plasmacytomas, which can cause bone pain, fractures, and a host of other skeletal complications. The malignant plasma cells also interfere with the production of healthy blood cells, leading to anemia, increased susceptibility to infections, and impaired blood clotting. The impact of multiple myeloma extends beyond the bones and bone marrow. The overproduction of abnormal antibodies, known as monoclonal proteins or M proteins, can have systemic effects. These proteins can accumulate in the blood and organs, causing damage to the kidneys, nerves, and other vital structures. The kidneys, in particular, are vulnerable to the toxic effects of M proteins, which can lead to renal impairment and, in severe cases, kidney failure.

The journey of living with multiple myeloma is often a long and arduous one, filled with physical, emotional, and psychological challenges. For patients and their loved ones, the diagnosis of multiple myeloma can be overwhelming and life-altering. The uncertainty of the future, the complexity of the disease, and the intensity of treatment regimens can take a toll on even the strongest individuals.

However, amidst the darkness, there is also a profound resilience and strength that emerges. Support networks, including family, friends, healthcare providers, and support groups, play a vital role in helping patients navigate the tumultuous waters of multiple myeloma. These networks provide not only practical assistance but also emotional solace and encouragement. They remind patients that they are not alone in their fight and that there is hope, even in the face of adversity. In recent years, advancements in research and treatment have brought new rays of hope to the multiple myeloma community. Innovative therapies, such as targeted therapies and immunotherapies, are transforming the landscape of multiple myeloma treatment. These treatments are designed to specifically target cancer cells while sparing healthy ones, offering a more personalized and less toxic approach to managing the disease. While the journey with multiple myeloma is undoubtedly challenging, it is also a testament to the resilience of the human spirit. Patients and their loved ones demonstrate remarkable courage and determination as they confront the myriad obstacles posed by this disease. Their stories of perseverance and hope serve as powerful reminders of the strength that lies within us all.

In summary, multiple myeloma is a formidable adversary, born from the intricate interplay of genetics and environmental factors. It disrupts the delicate balance of our bone marrow, leading to a cascade of health issues that can profoundly impact a patient's life. Yet, amidst the challenges, there is also hope, resilience, and a steadfast determination to overcome. Through the support of loved ones, advancements in research, and the indomitable human spirit, those affected by multiple myeloma continue to fight, inspire, and ultimately redefine what it means to live with this disease.

Symptoms and Diagnosis

Symptoms of Multiple Myeloma

Bone Pain and Fractures:

One of the most common and debilitating symptoms of multiple myeloma is bone pain. The malignant plasma cells proliferate within the bone marrow, causing the bones to weaken. This often leads to bone pain, particularly in the back, ribs, and hips. In severe cases, the weakened bones can fracture easily, even with minimal trauma, leading to what is known as pathological fractures.

Anemia:

As multiple myeloma progresses, it interferes with the production of healthy blood cells in the bone marrow. This disruption often leads to anemia, a condition characterized by a deficiency of red blood cells. Anemia can cause persistent fatigue, weakness, and shortness of breath, significantly affecting the patient's ability to carry out daily activities.

Frequent Infections: The overproduction of abnormal plasma cells in multiple myeloma compromises the immune system, making patients more susceptible to infections. Common infections include respiratory infections, urinary tract infections, and shingles. These infections can be recurrent and more severe than in individuals with a healthy immune system.

Hypercalcemia:

Multiple myeloma can cause the bones to release calcium into the bloodstream, leading to hypercalcemia, or elevated levels of calcium in the blood. Symptoms of hypercalcemia include nausea, vomiting, constipation, excessive thirst, frequent urination, confusion, and even kidney dysfunction. Severe hypercalcemia is a medical emergency and requires immediate attention.

Kidney Problems:

The abnormal proteins produced by myeloma cells, known as monoclonal proteins or M proteins, can damage the kidneys. This damage can impair kidney function, leading to symptoms such as increased urination, swelling in the legs and feet, and high blood pressure. In severe cases, it can lead to kidney failure, necessitating dialysis or kidney transplantation.

Neurological Symptoms:

In some cases, multiple myeloma can cause neurological symptoms. This can happen when the disease affects the bones of the spine, leading to compression of the spinal cord or nerves. Symptoms can include numbness or weakness in the limbs, difficulty walking, and in severe cases, loss of bowel or bladder control.

Diagnosis of Multiple Myeloma
Blood Tests:

Blood tests are a critical component of diagnosing multiple myeloma. These tests can reveal abnormalities such as high levels of calcium, anemia, and impaired kidney function. Specific tests like serum protein electrophoresis (SPEP) and immunofixation electrophoresis (IFE) are used to detect and measure monoclonal proteins (M proteins) in the blood, which are hallmarks of multiple myeloma.

Urine Tests:

Urine tests, particularly a 24-hour urine collection test, are used to detect Bence Jones proteins, a type of monoclonal light chain protein found in the urine of many multiple myeloma patients. The presence of these proteins can help confirm the diagnosis.

Bone Marrow Biopsy:

A definitive diagnosis of multiple myeloma often requires a bone marrow biopsy. During this procedure, a small sample of bone marrow is extracted, usually from the hip bone, and examined under a microscope. The biopsy can reveal the presence of abnormal plasma cells, providing a definitive diagnosis.

Imaging Tests:

Imaging tests such as X-rays, MRI (magnetic resonance imaging), CT (computed tomography) scans, and PET (positron emission tomography) scans are used to assess the extent of bone damage caused by multiple myeloma. These tests can identify areas of bone weakness, fractures, and the presence of plasmacytomas (tumors formed by myeloma cells).

Genetic Testing:

Genetic testing of bone marrow samples can provide valuable information about the specific genetic abnormalities associated with multiple myeloma. This information can help determine the prognosis and guide treatment decisions.

Treatment Options

The treatment of multiple myeloma, a type of cancer that affects plasma cells in the bone marrow, has seen significant advancements over the past few decades. The primary goals of treatment are to control the disease, manage symptoms, and improve the patient's quality of life. Treatment plans are typically personalized, considering the patient's overall health, stage of the disease, and specific genetic mutations associated with their myeloma.

Standard Treatment Options

1. Chemotherapy: Chemotherapy uses powerful drugs to kill rapidly dividing cancer cells. In multiple myeloma, chemotherapy is often used to reduce the number of malignant plasma cells in the bone marrow. Common chemotherapy drugs used include melphalan, cyclophosphamide, and vincristine. Chemotherapy can be administered orally or intravenously and is often combined with other treatments to enhance its effectiveness.

2. Targeted Therapy: Targeted therapy involves drugs that specifically target certain proteins or genes involved in the growth and survival of cancer cells. In multiple myeloma, targeted therapies such as proteasome inhibitors (e.g., bortezomib, carfilzomib) and monoclonal antibodies (e.g., daratumumab, elotuzumab) have shown significant efficacy. These drugs interfere with cancer cell mechanisms, leading to their destruction while minimizing damage to normal cells.

3. Immunotherapy: Immunotherapy leverages the body's immune system to fight cancer. In multiple myeloma, immunomodulatory drugs (IMiDs) like lenalidomide and pomalidomide boost the immune response against myeloma cells. Another form of immunotherapy is CAR-T cell therapy, where a patient's T-cells are genetically modified to target myeloma cells. Although still relatively new, CAR-T cell therapy has shown promise in patients with refractory multiple myeloma.

4. Stem Cell Transplantation: Stem cell transplantation, particularly autologous stem cell transplantation (ASCT), is a cornerstone treatment for multiple myeloma. In ASCT, a patient's own stem cells are harvested and stored. The patient then undergoes high-dose chemotherapy to eradicate myeloma cells, followed by the infusion of the stored stem cells to restore healthy bone marrow. This treatment can lead to prolonged remission in many patients.

Supportive and Symptom-Management Treatments
1. Bisphosphonates: Bisphosphonates, such as pamidronate and zoledronic acid, are used to strengthen bones and reduce bone pain and the risk of fractures. These drugs work by inhibiting bone resorption, a process that myeloma cells accelerate, leading to bone weakening.
2. Radiation Therapy: Radiation therapy uses high-energy beams to target and destroy cancer cells. In multiple myeloma, it is often used to relieve bone pain, shrink bone tumors, and treat spinal cord compression caused by plasmacytomas.
3. Pain Management: Managing pain is a crucial aspect of multiple myeloma treatment. A combination of medications, including analgesics, nonsteroidal anti-inflammatory drugs (NSAIDs), and opioids, may be used. Physical therapy and complementary therapies such as acupuncture and massage can also help alleviate pain.
4. Blood Transfusions: Anemia is a common complication of multiple myeloma. Blood transfusions can be necessary to increase red blood cell counts, thereby reducing fatigue and improving overall energy levels.

Clinical Trials and Emerging Therapies
1. Clinical Trials: Participation in clinical trials can provide access to new and experimental therapies that are not yet widely available. Clinical trials are crucial for advancing the understanding and treatment of multiple myeloma, and they offer patients the opportunity to receive cutting-edge treatments.
2. New Drug Developments: Research into multiple myeloma is continuously yielding new drugs and treatment combinations. Recent developments include next-generation proteasome inhibitors, novel monoclonal antibodies, and small-molecule inhibitors targeting specific pathways in myeloma cells. These emerging therapies hold the promise of improving outcomes and offering new hope for patients with resistant or relapsed multiple myeloma.

Integrated and Holistic Approaches
1. Nutrition and Diet: A balanced diet tailored to the needs of multiple myeloma patients can support overall health and treatment outcomes. Nutritional counseling can help manage side effects of treatment and maintain strength and energy.
2. Exercise: Regular physical activity, adapted to the patient's ability, can improve physical function, reduce fatigue, and enhance quality of life. Exercise programs should be designed in consultation with healthcare providers to ensure they are safe and beneficial.
3. Psychological Support: Living with multiple myeloma can be emotionally challenging. Psychological support through counseling, support groups, and stress management techniques is essential for mental well-being. Patients are encouraged to seek help for coping with anxiety, depression, and the emotional toll of their illness.

Chapter 2: The Role of Nutrition in Multiple Myeloma

How Diet Affects Multiple Myeloma

The relationship between diet and multiple myeloma is a deeply intricate and profoundly significant one. For those battling this complex cancer of the plasma cells, nutrition can be a powerful ally in managing symptoms, bolstering the immune system, and enhancing overall well-being. Understanding how diet affects multiple myeloma is crucial, not only for patients but also for their loved ones and caregivers who walk this challenging journey alongside them.

The Power of Nutrition in Multiple Myeloma

When confronted with the diagnosis of multiple myeloma, patients often find themselves grappling with a whirlwind of emotions and a barrage of medical information. Amidst this chaos, the role of diet might seem secondary, but it holds a pivotal place in the holistic management of the disease. A well-balanced, nutrient-rich diet can be a source of strength, providing the body with the essential tools it needs to fight back.

Boosting the Immune System: Multiple myeloma weakens the immune system, making patients more susceptible to infections. A diet rich in vitamins, minerals, and antioxidants can help fortify the immune system. Foods like fruits, vegetables, whole grains, nuts, and seeds are packed with these vital nutrients. Vitamin C, found in citrus fruits and leafy greens, and vitamin E, abundant in nuts and seeds, are particularly important for their immune-boosting properties. Omega-3 fatty acids, present in fatty fish like salmon and flaxseeds, have anti-inflammatory effects that can further support immune health.

Managing Treatment Side Effects: Chemotherapy and other treatments for multiple myeloma often come with a host of side effects, including nausea, fatigue, and loss of appetite. Here, diet plays a therapeutic role. Small, frequent meals and snacks can help maintain energy levels and manage nausea. Incorporating ginger and peppermint can alleviate nausea, while bland, easy-to-digest foods like bananas, rice, and applesauce can be gentle on the stomach. Staying hydrated is also crucial, as dehydration can exacerbate treatment side effects.

Maintaining Strength and Energy: Cancer and its treatment can lead to significant weight loss and muscle wasting. Ensuring adequate protein intake is essential for preserving muscle mass and maintaining strength. Lean meats, poultry, fish, eggs, dairy products, legumes, and soy products are excellent protein sources. Complex carbohydrates, such as whole grains, legumes, and starchy vegetables, provide sustained energy, helping patients combat fatigue and stay active.

Supporting Bone Health: Bone pain and fractures are common complications of multiple myeloma. Nutrients like calcium and vitamin D are critical for bone health. Dairy products, leafy greens, almonds, and fortified foods are good sources of calcium, while sunlight exposure and fortified foods help boost vitamin D levels. Additionally, magnesium and vitamin K, found in nuts, seeds, and green vegetables, play supportive roles in maintaining bone strength.

The Emotional Connection to Food

Food is more than just sustenance; it is an integral part of our emotional and cultural lives. For multiple myeloma patients, maintaining a positive relationship with food can be challenging yet profoundly rewarding. The act of preparing and enjoying a meal can bring comfort, a sense of normalcy, and moments of joy amidst the trials of cancer treatment.

The Comfort of Familiar Flavors: During tough times, familiar and favorite foods can provide emotional solace. While it's important to adhere to dietary recommendations, there's room for personal preferences and comfort foods in moderation. The smell of freshly baked bread, the warmth of a homemade soup, or the sweetness of a favorite dessert can uplift spirits and bring moments of happiness.

Sharing Meals with Loved Ones: Eating is often a communal activity, and sharing meals with family and friends can foster connection and support. Loved ones can play a crucial role by helping prepare nutritious meals, encouraging healthy eating habits, and simply being there to share in the experience. These shared moments can strengthen bonds and provide emotional nourishment.

The Journey to a Healthier Diet

Embarking on a healthier dietary journey is a process that requires patience, flexibility, and support. For multiple myeloma patients, it is essential to work closely with healthcare providers, including dietitians and nutritionists, to tailor a diet plan that meets their specific needs.

Setting Realistic Goals: Transitioning to a healthier diet doesn't happen overnight. Setting small, achievable goals can make the process manageable and less overwhelming. Simple steps, like incorporating more fruits and vegetables into daily meals, reducing processed foods, and staying hydrated, can make a significant difference over time.

Listening to the Body: Every individual's experience with multiple myeloma is unique, and so are their nutritional needs and tolerances. Patients should listen to their bodies and adjust their diets accordingly. If certain foods cause discomfort or side effects, it's important to discuss these issues with healthcare providers to find suitable alternatives.

Embracing Flexibility: Flexibility is key in managing diet during multiple myeloma. Treatment schedules, side effects, and overall health can vary, necessitating adjustments to meal plans. Being adaptable and open to change can help patients maintain a positive outlook and stay committed to their nutritional goals.

Foods to Include and Avoid

Foods to Include

1. Fruits and Vegetables: Fruits and vegetables are rich in vitamins, minerals, and antioxidants, which are vital for supporting the immune system and overall health. They are also high in fiber, which aids digestion and helps maintain a healthy weight. Some particularly beneficial options include:

- Berries (blueberries, strawberries, raspberries): High in antioxidants, which help fight free radicals and reduce inflammation.
- Leafy greens (spinach, kale, Swiss chard): Packed with vitamins A, C, and K, and folate, which support immune function and bone health.
- Cruciferous vegetables (broccoli, cauliflower, Brussels sprouts): Contain compounds that may have anti-cancer properties.
- Citrus fruits (oranges, lemons, grapefruits): Rich in vitamin C, which boosts the immune system and aids in iron absorption.

2. Whole Grains: Whole grains are an excellent source of complex carbohydrates, providing sustained energy and essential nutrients like fiber, B vitamins, and iron. Incorporating whole grains can help manage blood sugar levels and reduce fatigue. Examples include:

- Brown rice
- Quinoa
- Oats
- Whole wheat bread and pasta

3. Lean Proteins: Protein is essential for maintaining muscle mass and supporting the body's repair processes. Including a variety of lean protein sources can help meet the increased protein needs of multiple myeloma patients. Good options include:

- Poultry (chicken, turkey)
- Fish (salmon, trout, mackerel)
- Legumes (beans, lentils, chickpeas)
- Tofu and tempeh
- Low-fat dairy products (milk, yogurt, cheese)

4. Healthy Fats: Healthy fats are crucial for brain health, hormone production, and reducing inflammation. They should be included in moderation and sourced from:

- Olive oil and avocado oil
- Nuts and seeds (almonds, walnuts, chia seeds, flaxseeds)
- Avocados
- Fatty fish (salmon, sardines, mackerel)

5. Hydration: Staying hydrated is essential for all bodily functions, including nutrient transport and waste elimination. Drinking plenty of fluids, primarily water, is critical. Herbal teas and natural fruit-infused water can also be beneficial.

Foods to Avoid

1. Processed and Red Meats: Processed meats (such as bacon, sausage, and deli meats) and red meats have been linked to increased cancer risk due to their high levels of saturated fats and potential carcinogens formed during cooking. These should be limited or avoided.

2. High-Sugar Foods: Excessive sugar intake can lead to weight gain, increased inflammation, and potential interference with blood sugar control. Foods and beverages high in added sugars include:
- Sugary drinks (soda, energy drinks, sweetened teas)
- Sweets and desserts (candy, cakes, cookies, pastries)
- Sugary cereals

3. High-Sodium Foods: High sodium intake can exacerbate hypertension and kidney issues, which are common concerns for multiple myeloma patients. Foods to limit include:
- Processed and packaged foods (chips, crackers, instant noodles)
- Canned soups and vegetables with added salt
- Restaurant and fast food items

4. Fried and Fatty Foods: Fried and fatty foods are high in unhealthy fats, which can increase inflammation and the risk of cardiovascular disease. Examples include:
- Fried chicken and fish
- French fries and potato chips
- Baked goods made with hydrogenated oils

5. Alcohol: Alcohol can interfere with medication effectiveness and exacerbate liver and kidney problems. It can also weaken the immune system and contribute to dehydration. It's best to avoid or significantly limit alcohol consumption.

Breakfast Recipes

1. Blueberry Almond Smoothie

Ingredients:

- 1 cup unsweetened almond milk
- 1 cup fresh or frozen blueberries
- 1 ripe banana
- 1 tablespoon almond butter
- 1 tablespoon chia seeds
- 1 teaspoon honey (optional)
- 1/2 cup ice cubes (optional)

Instructions:

1. Place all ingredients into a blender.
2. Blend on high speed until smooth and creamy.
3. Pour into a glass and enjoy immediately.

Nutrition Info (per serving):

- Calories: 250
- Protein: 5g
- Carbohydrates: 40g
- Dietary Fiber: 8g
- Sugars: 22g
- Fat: 10g
- Saturated Fat: 1g
- Sodium: 150mg

Serves: 1 Cooking Time: 5 minutes

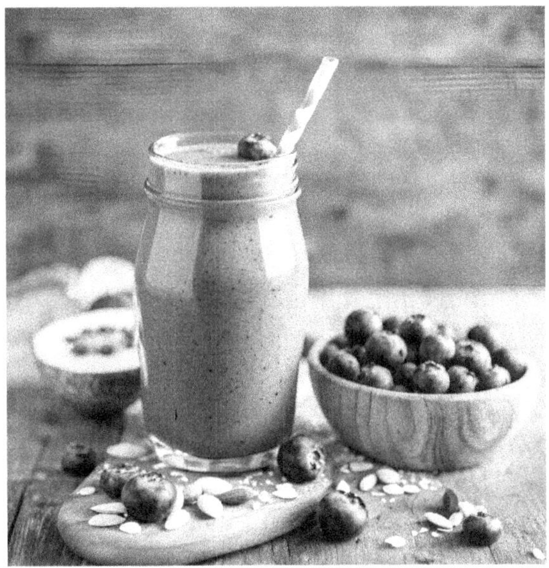

2. Berry Beet Smoothie

Ingredients:

- 1 small cooked beet, peeled and diced
- 1 cup mixed berries (strawberries, raspberries, blueberries)
- 1 cup unsweetened almond milk
- 1/2 cup plain Greek yogurt
- 1 tablespoon flaxseed meal
- 1 teaspoon maple syrup (optional)
- 1/2 cup ice cubes (optional)

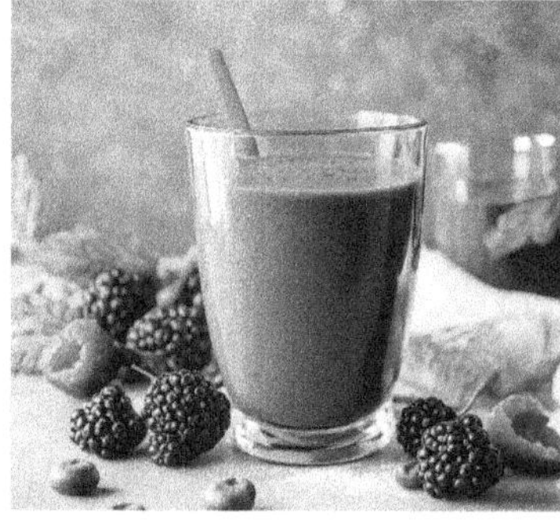

Instructions:

1. Add all ingredients to a blender.
2. Blend until smooth and well combined.
3. Pour into a glass and enjoy immediately.

Nutrition Info (per serving):

- Calories: 200   Protein: 8g   Carbohydrates: 35g   Dietary Fiber: 8g
- Sugars: 20g Fat: 5g Saturated Fat: 1.5g   Sodium: 120mg

Serves: 1 Cooking Time: 5 minutes

3. Oatmeal with Walnuts and Berries

Ingredients:

- 1 cup rolled oats
- 2 cups water or unsweetened almond milk
- 1/2 cup fresh or frozen mixed berries
- 1/4 cup chopped walnuts
- 1 tablespoon chia seeds
- 1 teaspoon cinnamon
- 1 teaspoon honey (optional)

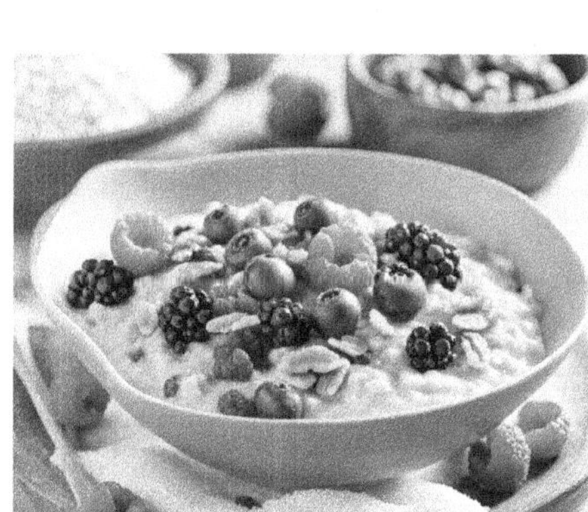

Instructions:

1. In a medium saucepan, bring the water or almond milk to a boil.
2. Add the rolled oats and reduce the heat to low. Cook, stirring occasionally, for about 5 minutes or until the oats are tender and have absorbed most of the liquid.
3. Stir in the cinnamon and chia seeds.
4. Serve topped with mixed berries, chopped walnuts, and a drizzle of honey if desired.

Nutrition Info (per serving):

- Calories: 350   Protein: 10g   Carbohydrates: 50g   Dietary Fiber: 9g
- Sugars: 10g Fat: 15g Saturated Fat: 1.5g Sodium: 5mg

Serves: 2 Cooking Time: 10 minutes

4. Creamy Buckwheat Porridge

Ingredients:

- 1 cup buckwheat groats
- 2 cups water
- 1 cup unsweetened almond milk
- 1 tablespoon ground flaxseed
- 1/2 teaspoon vanilla extract
- 1 tablespoon maple syrup
- Fresh fruit for topping (e.g., sliced bananas, berries)

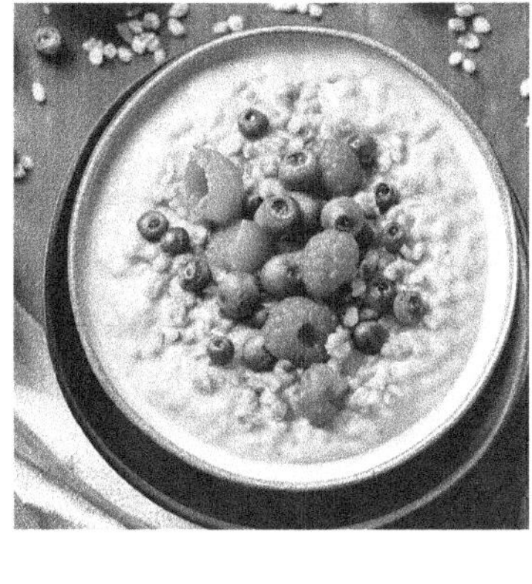

Instructions:

1. Rinse the buckwheat groats under cold water.
2. In a medium saucepan, bring the water to a boil. Add the buckwheat groats, reduce the heat to low, cover, and simmer for about 15 minutes or until the buckwheat is tender and the water is absorbed.
3. Stir in the almond milk, ground flaxseed, vanilla extract, and maple syrup. Cook for an additional 5 minutes, stirring frequently, until creamy.
4. Serve warm topped with fresh fruit.

Nutrition Info (per serving):

- Calories: 300 Protein: 8g Carbohydrates: 50g   Dietary Fiber: 8g
- Sugars: 10g   Fat: 7g   Saturated Fat: 0.5g Sodium: 10mg

Serves: 2 Cooking Time: 20 minutes

5. Millet Porridge with Honey and Nuts

Ingredients:

- 1 cup millet
- 2 cups water
- 1 cup unsweetened almond milk
- 1 tablespoon honey
- 1/4 cup chopped mixed nuts (almonds, walnuts, pecans)
- 1 teaspoon cinnamon
- Fresh fruit for topping (e.g., sliced apples, berries)

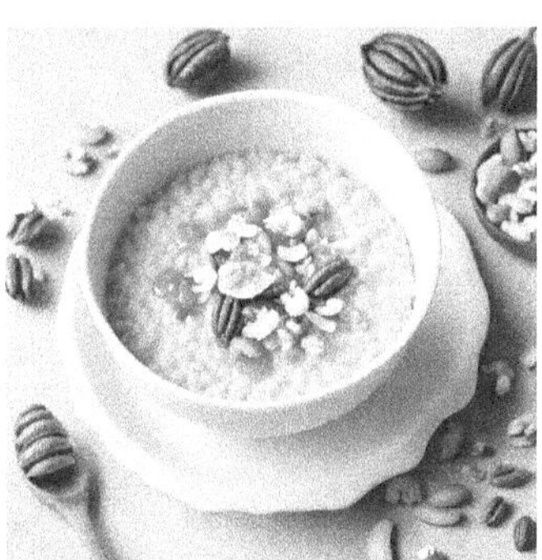

Instructions:

1. Rinse the millet under cold water.
2. In a medium saucepan, bring the water to a boil. Add the millet, reduce the heat to low, cover, and simmer for about 15 minutes or until the millet is tender and the water is absorbed.
3. Stir in the almond milk, honey, and cinnamon. Cook for an additional 5 minutes, stirring frequently, until creamy.
4. Serve warm topped with chopped nuts and fresh fruit.

Nutrition Info (per serving):

- Calories: 350   Protein: 9g Carbohydrates: 55g   Dietary Fiber: 7g
- Sugars: 12g   Fat: 12g Saturated Fat: 1g   Sodium: 5mg

Serves: 2 Cooking Time: 20 minutes

6. Soft Scrambled Eggs

Ingredients:

- 4 large eggs
- 2 tablespoons unsweetened almond milk
- 1 tablespoon olive oil
- 1 tablespoon chopped fresh chives (optional)
- 1/4 teaspoon turmeric (optional, for added anti-inflammatory benefits)

Instructions:

1. Crack the eggs into a bowl, add the almond milk, and whisk until well combined.
2. Heat the olive oil in a non-stick skillet over medium-low heat.
3. Pour in the egg mixture and cook slowly, stirring gently and continuously with a spatula, until the eggs are just set but still soft and creamy, about 4-5 minutes.
4. Serve immediately, garnished with chopped chives and a sprinkle of turmeric if desired.

Nutrition Info (per serving):

- Calories: 180
- Protein: 12g
- Carbohydrates: 2g
- Dietary Fiber: 0g
- Sugars: 0g
- Fat: 14g
- Saturated Fat: 3g
- Sodium: 70mg

Serves: 2 Cooking Time: 10 minutes

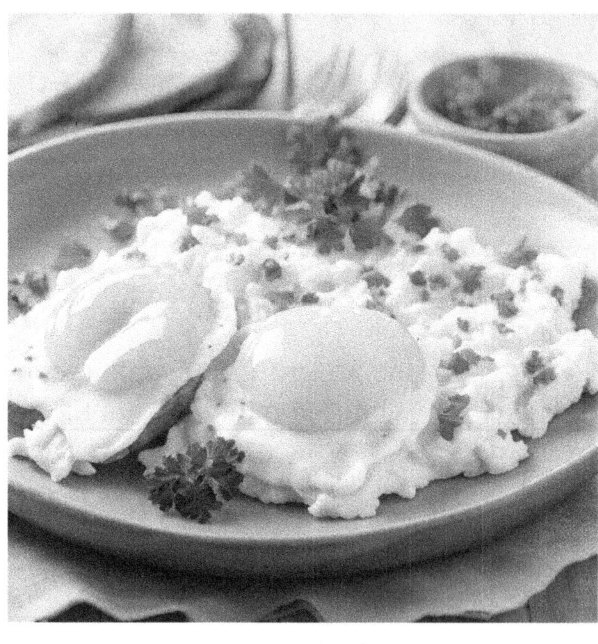

7. Egg White Omelette with Spinach

Ingredients:

- 4 large egg whites
- 1 cup fresh spinach leaves, chopped
- 1 tablespoon olive oil
- 1/4 cup diced tomatoes
- 1/4 cup chopped onions
- 1/2 teaspoon dried oregano

Instructions:

1. In a bowl, whisk the egg whites until slightly frothy.
2. Heat the olive oil in a non-stick skillet over medium heat.
3. Add the onions and cook until translucent, about 2-3 minutes.
4. Add the chopped spinach and tomatoes, and cook until the spinach is wilted, about 2 minutes.
5. Pour the egg whites over the vegetables and sprinkle with oregano. Cook until the egg whites are set, about 3-4 minutes, then fold the omelette in half.
6. Serve immediately.

Nutrition Info (per serving):

- Calories: 120
- Protein: 10g
- Carbohydrates: 5g
- Dietary Fiber: 2g
- Sugars: 3g
- Fat: 7g
- Saturated Fat: 1g
- Sodium: 150mg

Serves: 2 Cooking Time: 10 minutes

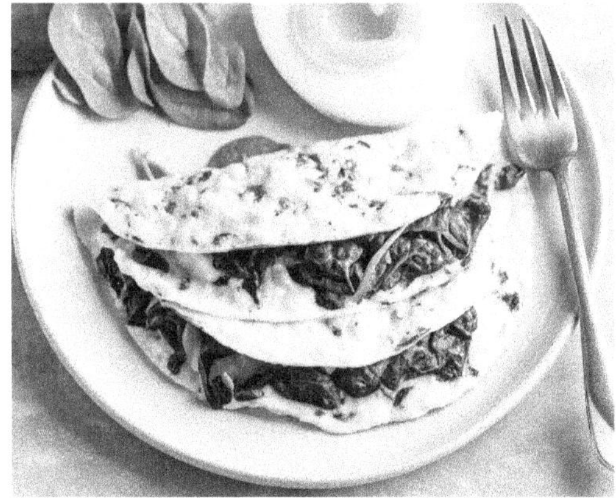

8. Silken Tofu Scramble

Ingredients:

- 1 block silken tofu, drained and crumbled
- 1 tablespoon olive oil
- 1/4 cup chopped red bell pepper
- 1/4 cup chopped green onions
- 1/2 teaspoon turmeric
- 1/2 teaspoon cumin
- 1 tablespoon nutritional yeast (optional, for a cheesy flavor)

Instructions:

1. Heat the olive oil in a non-stick skillet over medium heat.
2. Add the red bell pepper and green onions, and cook until softened, about 3 minutes.
3. Add the crumbled tofu, turmeric, and cumin, and cook for another 5-7 minutes, stirring frequently, until the tofu is heated through and slightly browned.
4. Stir in the nutritional yeast if using.
5. Serve immediately.

Nutrition Info (per serving):

- Calories: 150
- Protein: 12g
- Carbohydrates: 6g
- Dietary Fiber: 2g
- Sugars: 2g
- Fat: 10g
- Saturated Fat: 1.5g
- Sodium: 20mg

Serves: 2 Cooking Time: 10 minutes

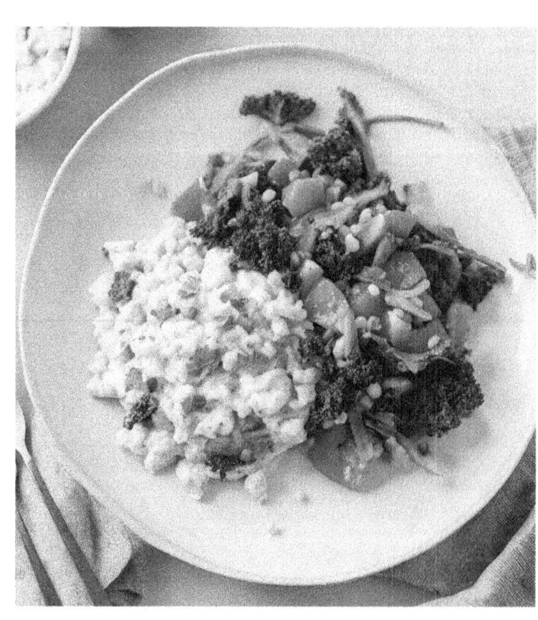

9. Poached Eggs over Asparagus

Ingredients:

- 4 large eggs
- 1 bunch asparagus, trimmed
- 1 tablespoon olive oil
- 1 tablespoon white vinegar
- 1 teaspoon lemon zest
- 1 tablespoon chopped fresh parsley

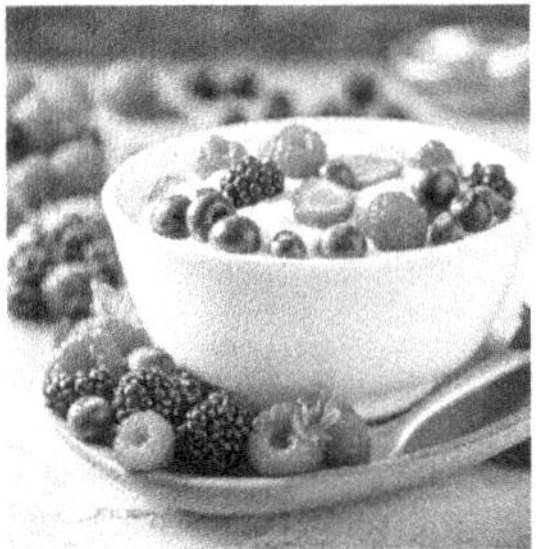

Instructions:

1. Preheat the oven to 400°F (200°C). Toss the asparagus with olive oil and spread on a baking sheet. Roast for 10-12 minutes until tender.
2. Meanwhile, bring a medium pot of water to a simmer. Add the vinegar.
3. Crack each egg into a small bowl, then gently slide it into the simmering water. Poach the eggs for 3-4 minutes, until the whites are set but the yolks are still runny.
4. Remove the eggs with a slotted spoon and drain on a paper towel.
5. Serve the poached eggs over the roasted asparagus, garnished with lemon zest and chopped parsley.

Nutrition Info (per serving):

- Calories: 200   Protein: 12g   Carbohydrates: 7g   Dietary Fiber: 3g   Sugars: 2g
- Fat: 15g   Saturated Fat: 3g   Sodium: 70mg

Serves: 2 Cooking Time: 15 minutes

10. Greek Yogurt with Mixed Berries

Ingredients:

- 1 cup plain Greek yogurt
- 1/2 cup fresh or frozen mixed berries (blueberries, strawberries, raspberries)
- 1 tablespoon honey
- 1 tablespoon chia seeds
- 1/4 teaspoon ground cinnamon

Instructions:

1. In a bowl, mix the Greek yogurt with honey and ground cinnamon.
2. Top with mixed berries and chia seeds.
3. Serve immediately.

Nutrition Info (per serving):

- Calories: 200   Protein: 14g   Carbohydrates: 28g   Dietary Fiber: 6g
- Sugars: 20g   Fat: 4g   Saturated Fat: 2g   Sodium: 70mg

Serves: 1 Cooking Time: 5 minutes

11. Kefir with Honey and Almonds

Ingredients:

- 1 cup plain kefir
- 1 tablespoon honey
- 2 tablespoons sliced almonds
- 1/4 teaspoon ground cinnamon

Instructions:

1. Pour the kefir into a glass or bowl.
2. Drizzle the honey over the kefir.
3. Sprinkle with sliced almonds and ground cinnamon.
4. Stir gently and enjoy immediately.

Nutrition Info (per serving):

- Calories: 210 Protein: 8g Carbohydrates: 24g Dietary Fiber: 2g
- Sugars: 18g Fat: 9g Saturated Fat: 1g Sodium: 110mg

Serves: 1 Cooking Time: 5 minutes

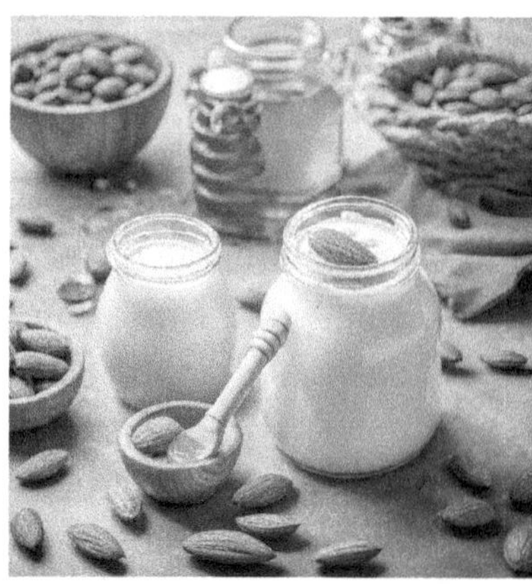

12. Yogurt Parfait with Muesli

Ingredients:

- 1 cup plain Greek yogurt
- 1/2 cup muesli
- 1/2 cup fresh mixed berries (blueberries, strawberries, raspberries)
- 1 tablespoon honey
- 1 tablespoon chia seeds

Instructions:

1. In a glass or bowl, layer half of the Greek yogurt.
2. Add a layer of muesli and then a layer of mixed berries.
3. Repeat the layers with the remaining yogurt, muesli, and berries.
4. Drizzle honey on top and sprinkle with chia seeds.
5. Serve immediately.

Nutrition Info (per serving):

- Calories: 300
- Protein: 14g
- Carbohydrates: 50g
- Dietary Fiber: 7g
- Sugars: 25g
- Fat: 8g
- Saturated Fat: 2g
- Sodium: 80mg

Serves: 1 Cooking Time: 5 minutes

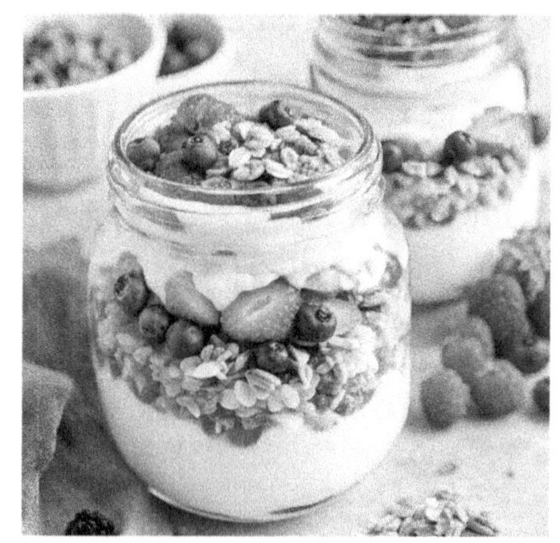

13. Avocado Toast with Sesame Seeds

Ingredients:

- 1 ripe avocado
- 2 slices whole grain bread
- 1 teaspoon sesame seeds
- 1 teaspoon lemon juice
- 1/4 teaspoon red pepper flakes (optional)

Instructions:

1. Toast the whole grain bread slices until golden brown.
2. While the bread is toasting, cut the avocado in half, remove the pit, and scoop the flesh into a bowl.
3. Mash the avocado with a fork and mix in the lemon juice.
4. Spread the mashed avocado evenly over the toasted bread slices.
5. Sprinkle sesame seeds and red pepper flakes (if using) on top.
6. Serve immediately.

Nutrition Info (per serving):

- Calories: 300   Protein: 7g   Carbohydrates: 30g   Dietary Fiber: 10g
- Sugars: 2g   Fat: 20g   Saturated Fat: 3g   Sodium: 150mg

Serves: 1 Cooking Time: 5 minutes

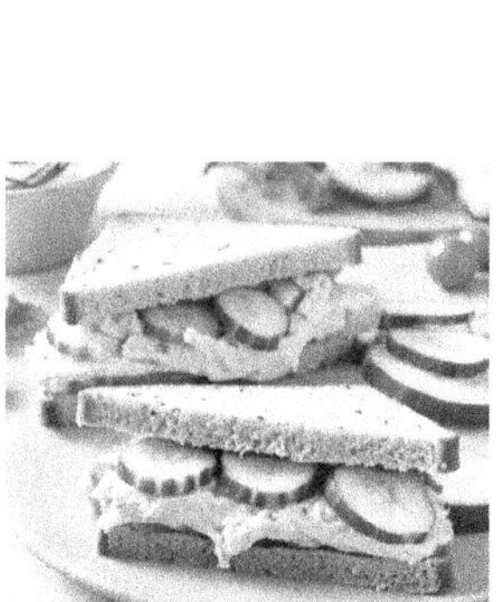

14. Hummus and Cucumber Sandwich

Ingredients:

- 4 slices whole grain bread
- 1 cup hummus
- 1 small cucumber, thinly sliced
- 1/4 cup grated carrots
- 1/4 cup alfalfa sprouts

Instructions:

1. Spread 1/4 cup of hummus on each slice of whole grain bread.
2. Layer cucumber slices, grated carrots, and alfalfa sprouts on two of the hummus-spread slices.
3. Top with the remaining slices of bread, hummus side down, to form sandwiches.
4. Cut each sandwich in half and serve immediately.

Nutrition Info (per serving):

- Calories: 350 Protein: 12g   Carbohydrates: 48g
- Dietary Fiber: 10g   Sugars: 5g   Fat: 12g
- Saturated Fat: 2g
- Sodium: 400mg

Serves: 2 Cooking Time: 10 minutes

15. Banana Oat Pancakes

Ingredients:

- 1 cup rolled oats
- 2 ripe bananas
- 2 large eggs
- 1/2 teaspoon baking powder
- 1/2 teaspoon vanilla extract
- 1/2 teaspoon ground cinnamon
- 1 tablespoon coconut oil (for cooking)
- Fresh fruit for topping (e.g., berries, sliced bananas)

Instructions:

1. Place the rolled oats in a blender and blend until they become a fine flour.
2. Add the bananas, eggs, baking powder, vanilla extract, and ground cinnamon to the blender. Blend until smooth.
3. Heat a non-stick skillet over medium heat and add a small amount of coconut oil.
4. Pour about 1/4 cup of the batter into the skillet for each pancake. Cook until bubbles form on the surface and the edges look set, about 2-3 minutes.
5. Flip the pancakes and cook for another 2-3 minutes, until golden brown and cooked through.
6. Repeat with the remaining batter, adding more coconut oil to the skillet as needed.
7. Serve the pancakes topped with fresh fruit.

Nutrition Info (per serving):

- Calories: 250
- Protein: 8g
- Carbohydrates: 40g
- Dietary Fiber: 6g
- Sugars: 12g
- Fat: 8g
- Saturated Fat: 4g
- Sodium: 150mg

Serves: 2 Cooking Time: 20 minutes

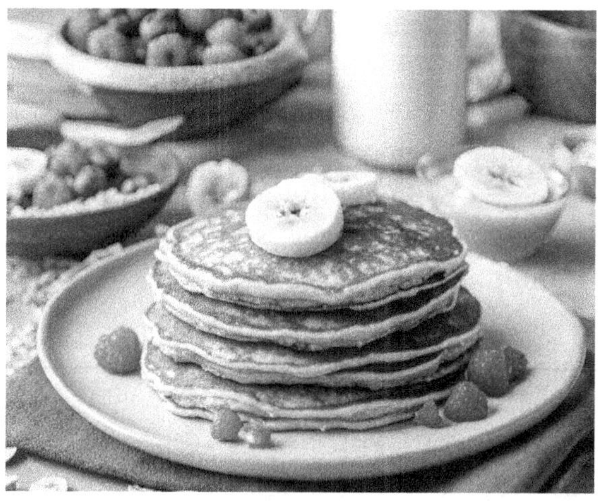

16. Fruit Salad with Mint

Ingredients:

- 1 cup strawberries, hulled and quartered
- 1 cup blueberries
- 1 cup diced pineapple
- 1 cup diced kiwi
- 1 tablespoon fresh mint leaves, finely chopped
- 1 tablespoon honey
- 1 tablespoon fresh lime juice

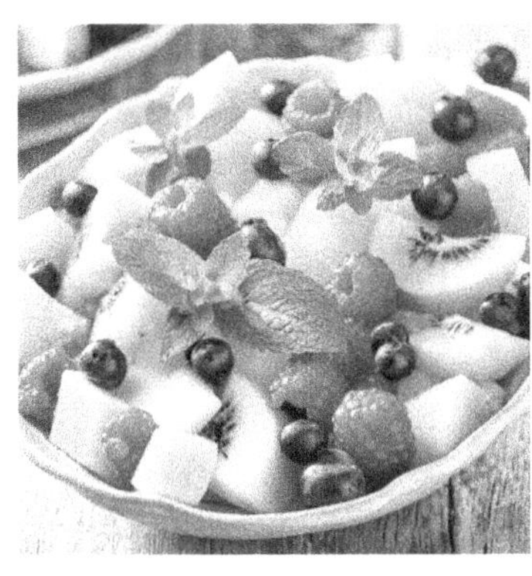

Instructions:

1. In a large bowl, combine the strawberries, blueberries, pineapple, and kiwi.
2. In a small bowl, mix the honey and lime juice until well combined.
3. Pour the honey-lime mixture over the fruit and gently toss to coat.
4. Sprinkle the chopped mint leaves over the fruit salad and toss again.
5. Serve immediately or refrigerate until ready to serve.

Nutrition Info (per serving):

- Calories: 100   Protein: 1g   Carbohydrates: 25g   Dietary Fiber: 4g
- Sugars: 20g   Fat: 0g   Saturated Fat: 0g   Sodium: 5mg

Serves: 4 Cooking Time: 10 minutes

17. Melon and Prosciutto Plate

Ingredients:

- 1 small cantaloupe, peeled, seeded, and sliced
- 1 small honeydew melon, peeled, seeded, and sliced
- 6 slices prosciutto
- 1 tablespoon fresh mint leaves, finely chopped

Instructions:

1. Arrange the cantaloupe and honeydew melon slices on a serving platter.
2. Drape the prosciutto slices over the melon.
3. Sprinkle the chopped mint leaves over the top.
4. Serve immediately.

Nutrition Info (per serving):

- Calories: 120
- Protein: 7g
- Carbohydrates: 14g
- Dietary Fiber: 1g
- Sugars: 12g
- Fat: 5g
- Saturated Fat: 2g
- Sodium: 400mg

Serves: 4 Cooking Time: 10 minutes

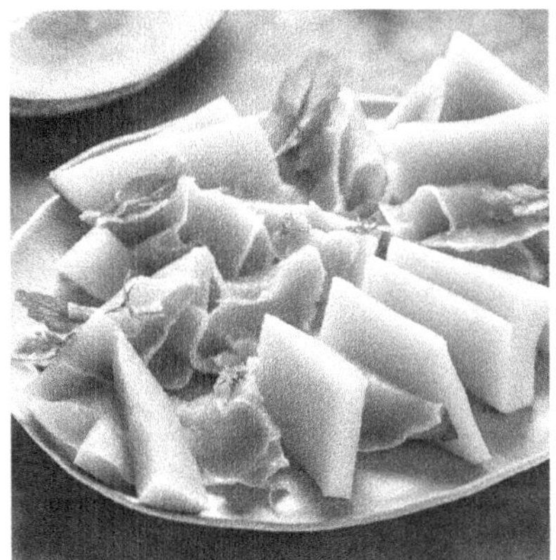

18. Coconut Yogurt and Mango

Ingredients:

- 1 cup coconut yogurt
- 1 ripe mango, peeled and diced
- 1 tablespoon unsweetened shredded coconut
- 1 teaspoon chia seeds

Instructions:

1. Divide the coconut yogurt between two bowls.
2. Top each bowl with diced mango.
3. Sprinkle with shredded coconut and chia seeds.
4. Serve immediately.

Nutrition Info (per serving):

- Calories: 200
- Protein: 3g
- Carbohydrates: 28g
- Dietary Fiber: 4g
- Sugars: 20g
- Fat: 9g
- Saturated Fat: 7g
- Sodium: 30mg

Serves: 2 Cooking Time: 5 minutes

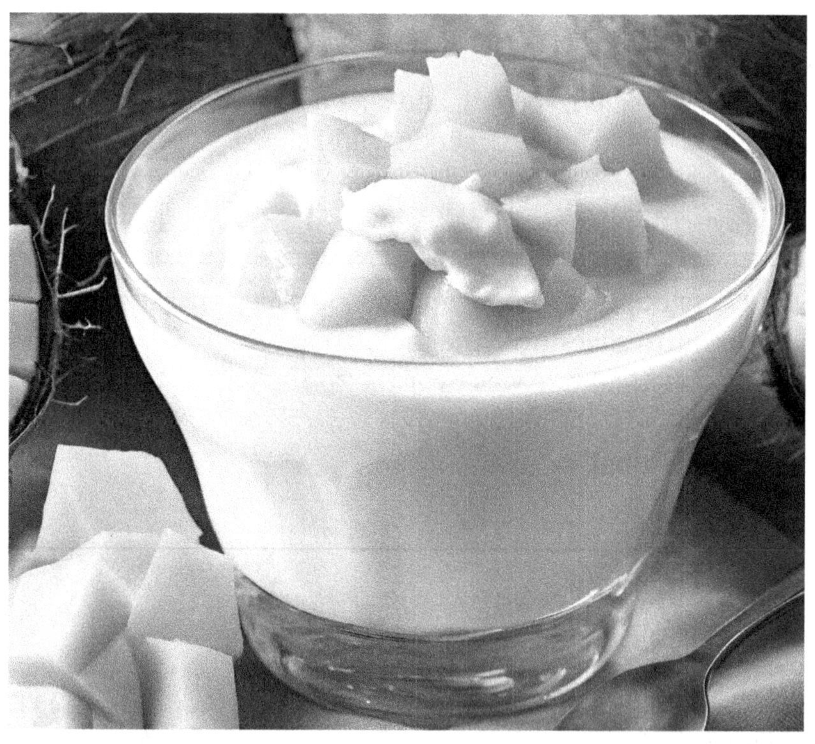

19. Almond Flour Waffles

Ingredients:

- 1 1/2 cups almond flour
- 1/2 teaspoon baking soda
- 1/4 teaspoon ground cinnamon
- 3 large eggs
- 1/4 cup unsweetened almond milk
- 1 tablespoon honey
- 1 teaspoon vanilla extract
- 1 tablespoon coconut oil, melted

Instructions:

1. Preheat your waffle iron according to the manufacturer's instructions.
2. In a large bowl, whisk together the almond flour, baking soda, and ground cinnamon.
3. In another bowl, whisk together the eggs, almond milk, honey, vanilla extract, and melted coconut oil.
4. Pour the wet ingredients into the dry ingredients and mix until well combined.
5. Grease the waffle iron with a bit of coconut oil. Pour the batter onto the waffle iron and cook until golden brown and crispy, about 3-4 minutes.
6. Serve immediately with your favorite toppings such as fresh fruit or a drizzle of honey.

Nutrition Info (per serving):

- Calories: 250
- Protein: 10g
- Carbohydrates: 15g
- Dietary Fiber: 3g
- Sugars: 6g
- Fat: 18g
- Saturated Fat: 5g
- Sodium: 180mg

Serves: 4 Cooking Time: 15 minutes

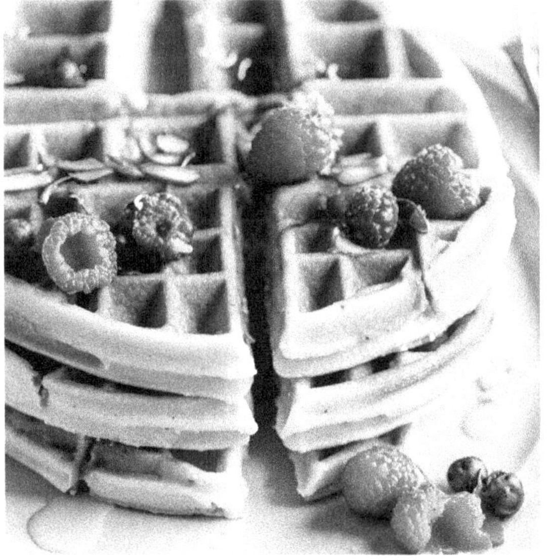

20. Cottage Cheese Pancakes

Ingredients:

- 1 cup cottage cheese
- 3 large eggs
- 1/2 cup oat flour
- 1 tablespoon honey
- 1/2 teaspoon baking powder
- 1/4 teaspoon ground cinnamon
- 1 tablespoon coconut oil (for cooking)

Instructions:

1. In a blender, combine the cottage cheese, eggs, oat flour, honey, baking powder, and ground cinnamon. Blend until smooth.
2. Heat a non-stick skillet over medium heat and add a small amount of coconut oil.
3. Pour about 1/4 cup of the batter into the skillet for each pancake. Cook until bubbles form on the surface and the edges look set, about 2-3 minutes.
4. Flip the pancakes and cook for another 2-3 minutes, until golden brown and cooked through.
5. Repeat with the remaining batter, adding more coconut oil to the skillet as needed.
6. Serve the pancakes warm, with fresh fruit or a drizzle of honey if desired.

Nutrition Info (per serving):

- Calories: 200
- Protein: 12g
- Carbohydrates: 20g
- Dietary Fiber: 2g
- Sugars: 6g
- Fat: 8g
- Saturated Fat: 4g
- Sodium: 300mg

Serves: 4 Cooking Time: 15 minutes

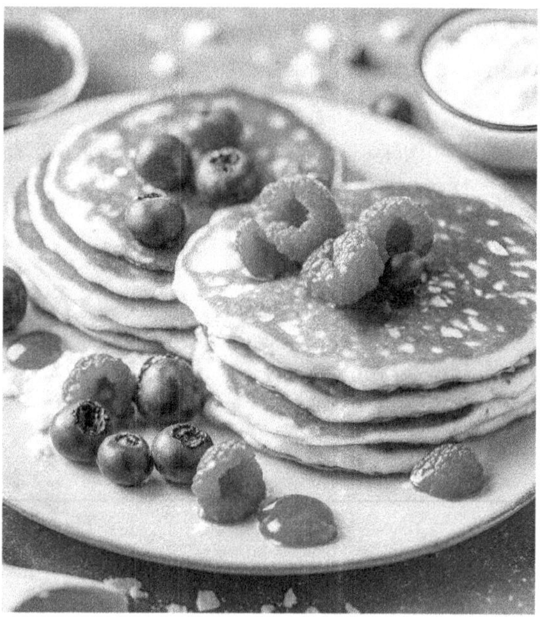

21. Buckwheat Pancakes with Honey

Ingredients:

- 1 cup buckwheat flour
- 1 teaspoon baking powder
- 1/2 teaspoon ground cinnamon
- 1 large egg
- 1 cup unsweetened almond milk
- 1 tablespoon honey
- 1 tablespoon coconut oil (for cooking)
- Additional honey for serving

Instructions:

1. In a large bowl, mix the buckwheat flour, baking powder, and ground cinnamon.
2. In another bowl, whisk together the egg, almond milk, and honey.
3. Pour the wet ingredients into the dry ingredients and mix until just combined.
4. Heat a non-stick skillet over medium heat and add a small amount of coconut oil.
5. Pour about 1/4 cup of the batter into the skillet for each pancake. Cook until bubbles form on the surface and the edges look set, about 2-3 minutes.
6. Flip the pancakes and cook for another 2-3 minutes, until golden brown and cooked through.
7. Repeat with the remaining batter, adding more coconut oil to the skillet as needed.
8. Serve the pancakes warm with additional honey drizzled on top.

Nutrition Info (per serving):

- Calories: 220
- Protein: 6g
- Carbohydrates: 35g
- Dietary Fiber: 5g
- Sugars: 10g
- Fat: 7g
- Saturated Fat: 4g
- Sodium: 100mg

Serves: 4 Cooking Time: 20 minutes

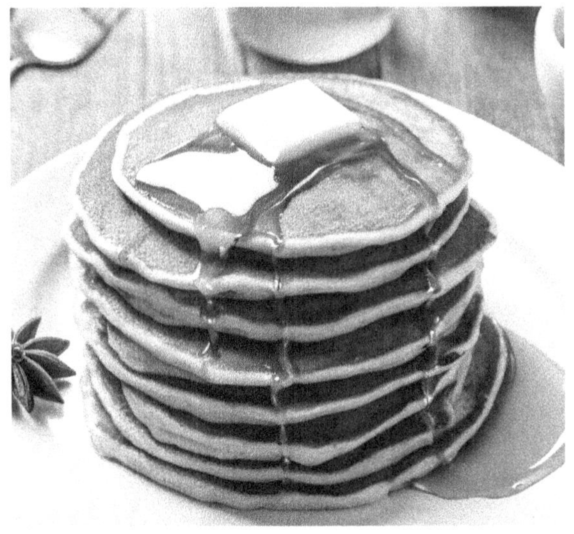

22. Steamed Vegetable Medley

Ingredients:

- 1 cup broccoli florets
- 1 cup cauliflower florets
- 1 cup baby carrots
- 1 cup green beans, trimmed
- 1 tablespoon olive oil
- 1 teaspoon lemon juice
- 1 tablespoon chopped fresh parsley

Instructions:

1. Fill a large pot with about an inch of water and bring to a boil. Place a steamer basket in the pot.
2. Add the broccoli, cauliflower, baby carrots, and green beans to the steamer basket. Cover and steam for about 5-7 minutes, until the vegetables are tender.
3. Transfer the steamed vegetables to a serving bowl.
4. Drizzle with olive oil and lemon juice, and sprinkle with chopped parsley.
5. Toss gently to combine and serve immediately.

Nutrition Info (per serving):

- Calories: 100
- Protein: 3g
- Carbohydrates: 15g
- Dietary Fiber: 5g
- Sugars: 5g
- Fat: 5g
- Saturated Fat: 0.5g
- Sodium: 50mg

Serves: 4 Cooking Time: 10 minutes

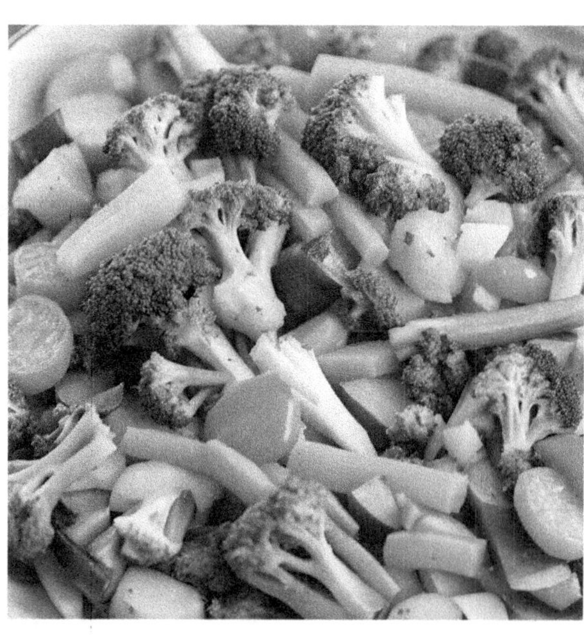

23. Sautéed Mushrooms

Ingredients:
- 2 cups sliced mushrooms (e.g., cremini, button, or shiitake)
- 1 tablespoon olive oil
- 1 teaspoon minced garlic
- 1 tablespoon fresh thyme leaves
- 1 teaspoon balsamic vinegar

Instructions:
1. Heat the olive oil in a large skillet over medium heat.
2. Add the minced garlic and cook for about 1 minute until fragrant.
3. Add the sliced mushrooms and cook, stirring occasionally, for about 5-7 minutes, until the mushrooms are tender and browned.
4. Stir in the fresh thyme leaves and balsamic vinegar.
5. Cook for an additional 1-2 minutes, until the mushrooms are well coated and the vinegar has reduced slightly.
6. Serve immediately.

Nutrition Info (per serving):
- Calories: 90
- Protein: 3g
- Carbohydrates: 5g
- Dietary Fiber: 2g
- Sugars: 2g
- Fat: 7g
- Saturated Fat: 1g
- Sodium: 10mg

Serves: 2 Cooking Time: 10 minutes

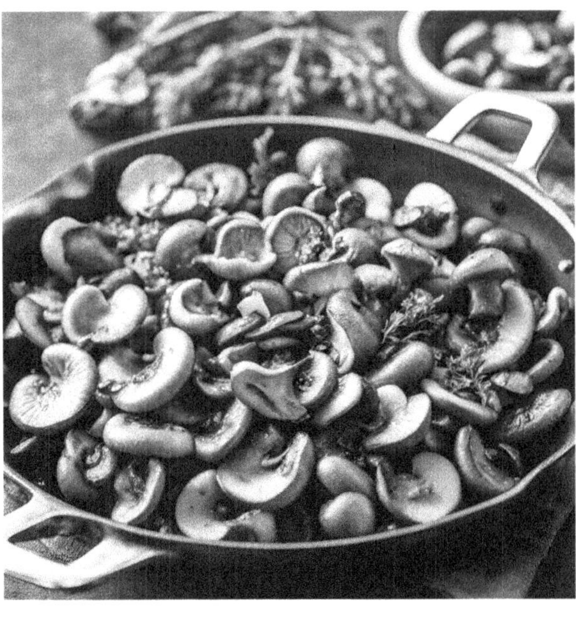

24. Whole Grain Waffles

Ingredients:

- 1 cup whole wheat flour
- 1/2 cup rolled oats
- 1 teaspoon baking powder
- 1/2 teaspoon ground cinnamon
- 1 large egg
- 1 cup unsweetened almond milk
- 1 tablespoon honey
- 2 tablespoons coconut oil, melted
- 1 teaspoon vanilla extract

Instructions:

1. Preheat your waffle iron according to the manufacturer's instructions.
2. In a large bowl, combine the whole wheat flour, rolled oats, baking powder, and ground cinnamon.
3. In another bowl, whisk together the egg, almond milk, honey, melted coconut oil, and vanilla extract.
4. Pour the wet ingredients into the dry ingredients and mix until just combined.
5. Grease the waffle iron with a bit of coconut oil. Pour the batter onto the waffle iron and cook until golden brown and crispy, about 3-4 minutes.
6. Serve immediately with your favorite toppings such as fresh fruit or a drizzle of honey.

Nutrition Info (per serving):

- Calories: 250
- Protein: 8g
- Carbohydrates: 35g
- Dietary Fiber: 6g
- Sugars: 8g
- Fat: 10g
- Saturated Fat: 4g
- Sodium: 150mg

Serves: 4 Cooking Time: 15 minutes

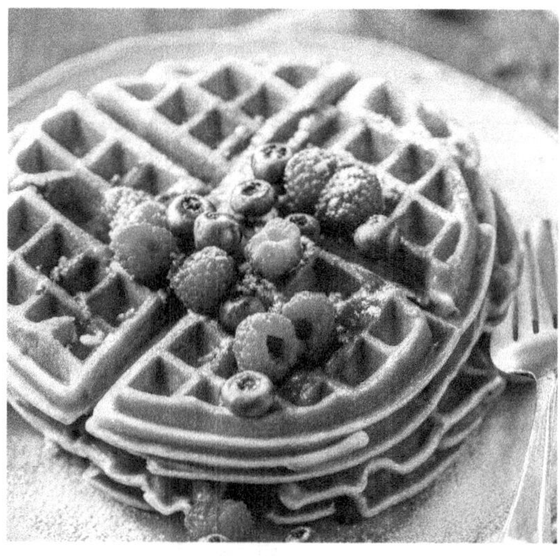

Fish Recipes

1. Baked Salmon with Dill and Lemon

Ingredients:

- 4 salmon fillets (about 6 ounces each)
- 1 lemon, thinly sliced
- 1 tablespoon fresh dill, chopped
- 2 tablespoons olive oil
- 2 garlic cloves, minced
- 1/2 teaspoon paprika

Instructions:

1. Preheat the oven to 375°F (190°C).
2. Place the salmon fillets on a baking sheet lined with parchment paper.
3. In a small bowl, mix the olive oil, minced garlic, and paprika.
4. Brush the olive oil mixture over the salmon fillets.
5. Lay lemon slices on top of the salmon fillets.
6. Sprinkle the chopped dill over the lemon slices.
7. Bake in the preheated oven for 15-20 minutes, or until the salmon is cooked through and flakes easily with a fork.
8. Serve immediately.

Nutrition Info (per serving):

- Calories: 350
- Protein: 34g
- Carbohydrates: 2g
- Dietary Fiber: 0g
- Sugars: 0g
- Fat: 22g
- Saturated Fat: 4g
- Sodium: 70mg

Serves: 4 Cooking Time: 20 minutes

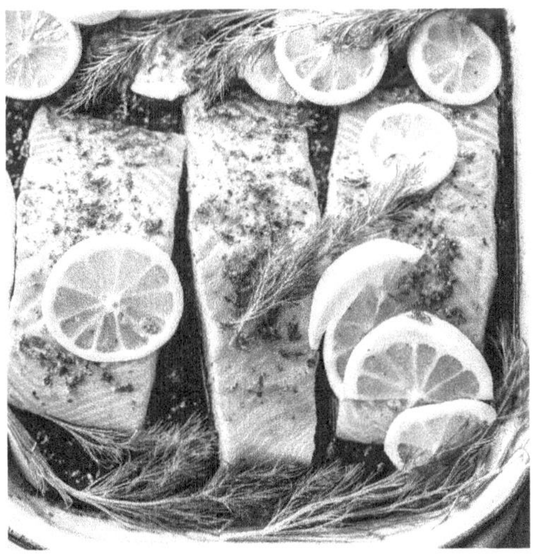

2. Grilled Tuna Steaks with Olive Tapenade

Ingredients:

- 4 tuna steaks (about 6 ounces each)
- 2 tablespoons olive oil
- 1 tablespoon lemon juice
- 1 teaspoon dried oregano
- 1/2 cup black olives, pitted and chopped
- 1/4 cup sun-dried tomatoes, chopped
- 2 tablespoons capers, rinsed and drained
- 1 garlic clove, minced
- 1 tablespoon fresh parsley, chopped

Instructions:

1. In a small bowl, mix 1 tablespoon of olive oil, lemon juice, and dried oregano.
2. Brush the mixture over the tuna steaks and let them marinate for about 15 minutes.
3. Preheat the grill to medium-high heat.
4. Grill the tuna steaks for about 3-4 minutes on each side, or until desired doneness.
5. In another bowl, mix the chopped olives, sun-dried tomatoes, capers, minced garlic, and remaining olive oil to make the tapenade.
6. Serve the grilled tuna steaks topped with the olive tapenade and sprinkled with fresh parsley.

Nutrition Info (per serving):

- Calories: 320   Protein: 36g   Carbohydrates: 3g   Dietary Fiber: 1g
- Sugars: 1g   Fat: 18g   Saturated Fat: 3g   Sodium: 300mg

Serves: 4 Cooking Time: 15 minutes (plus 15 minutes marinating time)

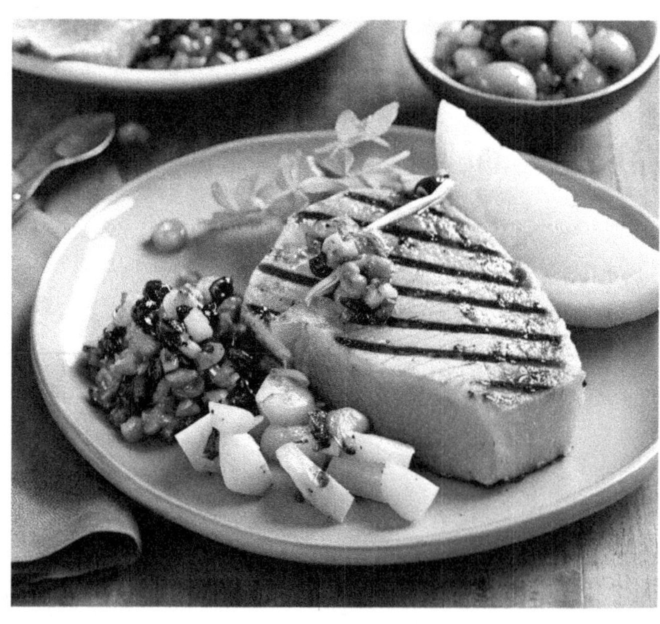

3. Poached Cod in Tomato Broth

Ingredients:

- 4 cod fillets (about 6 ounces each)
- 1 tablespoon olive oil
- 1 medium onion, chopped
- 2 garlic cloves, minced
- 1 can (14.5 ounces) diced tomatoes, with juice
- 1 cup low-sodium vegetable broth
- 1 teaspoon dried basil
- 1 teaspoon dried oregano
- 1/4 teaspoon crushed red pepper flakes (optional)
- 1 tablespoon fresh basil, chopped (for garnish)

Instructions:

1. Heat the olive oil in a large skillet over medium heat.
2. Add the chopped onion and cook until softened, about 5 minutes.
3. Add the minced garlic and cook for another 1 minute.
4. Stir in the diced tomatoes with juice, vegetable broth, dried basil, dried oregano, and crushed red pepper flakes if using. Bring to a simmer.
5. Add the cod fillets to the skillet, spooning some of the tomato broth over the top.
6. Cover and cook for about 10-12 minutes, or until the cod is opaque and flakes easily with a fork.
7. Serve the poached cod in bowls with the tomato broth and garnish with chopped fresh basil.

Nutrition Info (per serving):

- Calories: 220
- Protein: 30g
- Carbohydrates: 10g
- Dietary Fiber: 2g
- Sugars: 6g
- Fat: 6g
- Saturated Fat: 1g
- Sodium: 150mg

Serves: 4 Cooking Time: 25 minutes

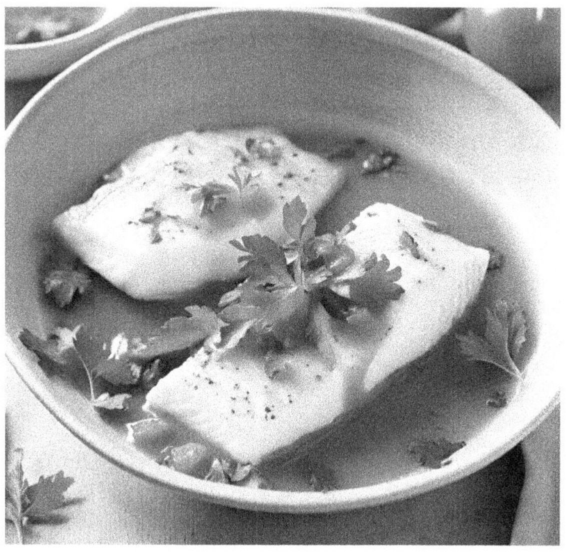

4. Herb-Crusted Tilapia

Ingredients:

- 4 tilapia fillets (about 6 ounces each)
- 1 cup whole wheat breadcrumbs
- 2 tablespoons fresh parsley, chopped
- 2 tablespoons fresh basil, chopped
- 1 tablespoon fresh thyme, chopped
- 2 garlic cloves, minced
- 1 lemon, zested and juiced
- 2 tablespoons olive oil
- 1 egg, beaten

Instructions:

1. Preheat the oven to 375°F (190°C). Line a baking sheet with parchment paper.
2. In a bowl, mix the breadcrumbs, parsley, basil, thyme, minced garlic, lemon zest, and 1 tablespoon of olive oil.
3. Brush the tilapia fillets with the beaten egg.
4. Press the breadcrumb mixture onto both sides of each fillet.
5. Place the fillets on the prepared baking sheet.
6. Drizzle with the remaining olive oil.
7. Bake for 15-20 minutes, until the fish is golden and flakes easily with a fork.
8. Squeeze lemon juice over the top before serving.

Nutrition Info (per serving):

- Calories: 300
- Protein: 28g
- Carbohydrates: 15g
- Dietary Fiber: 2g
- Sugars: 1g
- Fat: 15g
- Saturated Fat: 2.5g
- Sodium: 90mg

Serves: 4 Cooking Time: 25 minutes

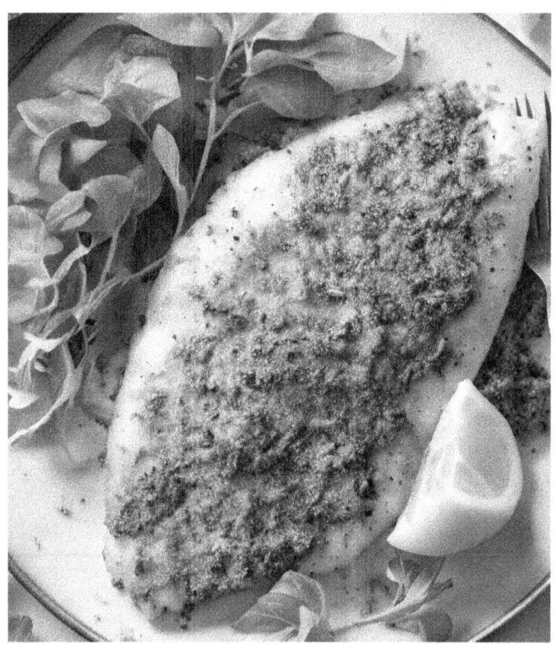

5. Shrimp and Quinoa Salad

Ingredients:

- 1 cup quinoa, rinsed
- 2 cups water
- 1 pound large shrimp, peeled and deveined
- 2 tablespoons olive oil
- 1 cup cherry tomatoes, halved
- 1 cucumber, diced
- 1/4 cup red onion, finely chopped
- 1/4 cup fresh parsley, chopped
- 1 lemon, juiced
- 1 teaspoon dried oregano

Instructions:

1. In a medium saucepan, bring water to a boil. Add the quinoa, reduce heat to low, cover, and simmer for about 15 minutes, until water is absorbed and quinoa is tender. Fluff with a fork and let cool.
2. Heat 1 tablespoon of olive oil in a large skillet over medium heat. Add the shrimp and cook until pink and opaque, about 2-3 minutes per side. Remove from heat and let cool.
3. In a large bowl, combine the cooled quinoa, shrimp, cherry tomatoes, cucumber, red onion, and parsley.
4. In a small bowl, whisk together the lemon juice, remaining olive oil, and oregano. Pour over the salad and toss to coat.
5. Serve immediately or refrigerate until ready to serve.

Nutrition Info (per serving):

- Calories: 350
- Protein: 28g
- Carbohydrates: 28g
- Dietary Fiber: 4g
- Sugars: 3g
- Fat: 14g
- Saturated Fat: 2g
- Sodium: 210mg

Serves: 4 Cooking Time: 25 minutes

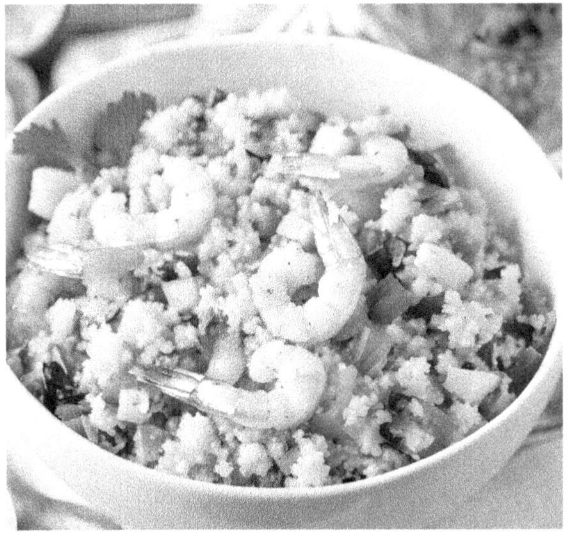

6. Mackerel Pate

Ingredients:

- 1 cup smoked mackerel, skin removed and flaked
- 1/2 cup Greek yogurt
- 1 tablespoon lemon juice
- 1 tablespoon fresh dill, chopped
- 1 tablespoon capers, rinsed and drained
- 1/2 teaspoon Dijon mustard
- 1 small shallot, finely chopped

Instructions:

1. In a food processor, combine the smoked mackerel, Greek yogurt, lemon juice, dill, capers, Dijon mustard, and shallot.
2. Blend until smooth and creamy.
3. Transfer to a serving dish and refrigerate for at least 1 hour before serving.
4. Serve with whole grain crackers or vegetable sticks.

Nutrition Info (per serving):

- Calories: 150
- Protein: 14g
- Carbohydrates: 3g
- Dietary Fiber: 0g
- Sugars: 1g
- Fat: 9g
- Saturated Fat: 2.5g
- Sodium: 150mg

Serves: 4 Cooking Time: 10 minutes (plus 1 hour chilling time)

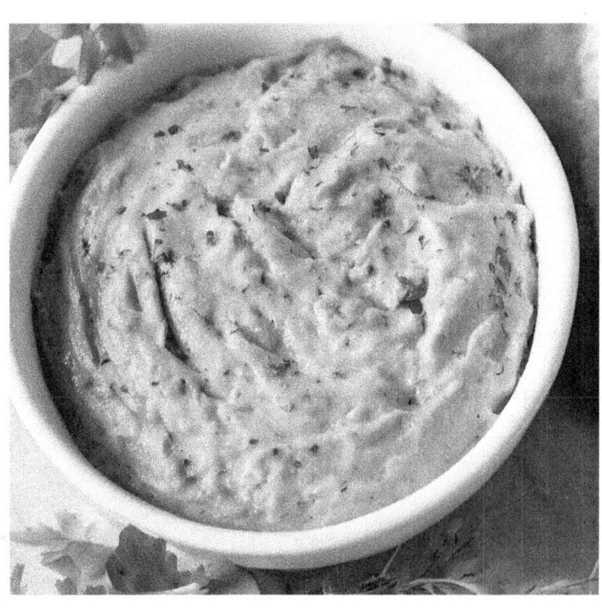

7. Trout Almondine

Ingredients:

- 4 trout fillets (about 6 ounces each)
- 1/2 cup sliced almonds
- 2 tablespoons olive oil
- 2 tablespoons fresh lemon juice
- 2 tablespoons fresh parsley, chopped
- 2 garlic cloves, minced

Instructions:

1. Preheat the oven to 375°F (190°C). Line a baking sheet with parchment paper.
2. Place the trout fillets on the prepared baking sheet.
3. In a small bowl, mix the olive oil, lemon juice, and minced garlic.
4. Brush the olive oil mixture over the trout fillets.
5. Sprinkle the sliced almonds evenly over the top of each fillet.
6. Bake for 15-20 minutes, until the trout is cooked through and the almonds are golden brown.
7. Garnish with chopped parsley and serve immediately.

Nutrition Info (per serving):

- Calories: 350
- Protein: 30g
- Carbohydrates: 4g
- Dietary Fiber: 2g
- Sugars: 1g
- Fat: 22g
- Saturated Fat: 3.5g
- Sodium: 70mg

Serves: 4 Cooking Time: 20 minutes

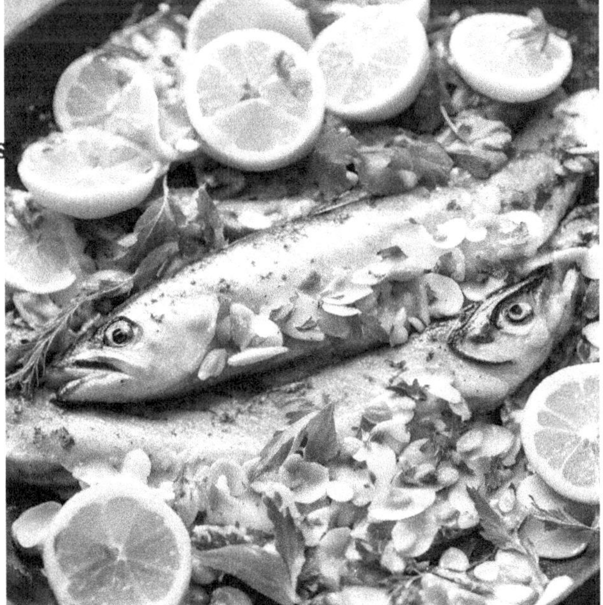

8. Haddock in Parchment with Vegetables
Ingredients:
- 4 haddock fillets (about 6 ounces each)
- 1 zucchini, thinly sliced
- 1 yellow squash, thinly sliced
- 1 red bell pepper, thinly sliced
- 1 carrot, julienned
- 2 tablespoons olive oil
- 1 lemon, thinly sliced
- 1 tablespoon fresh thyme leaves

Instructions:
1. Preheat the oven to 400°F (200°C).
2. Cut 4 large pieces of parchment paper, about 12 inches square each.
3. In a bowl, toss the zucchini, yellow squash, red bell pepper, and carrot with 1 tablespoon of olive oil and fresh thyme leaves.
4. Place one haddock fillet in the center of each piece of parchment paper.
5. Divide the vegetable mixture evenly among the parchment squares, placing the vegetables on top of the fish.
6. Top each fillet with a few lemon slices.
7. Drizzle the remaining olive oil over the fish and vegetables.
8. Fold the parchment paper over the fish and vegetables, crimping the edges to seal completely.
9. Place the parchment packets on a baking sheet and bake for 20-25 minutes, until the fish is opaque and cooked through.
10. Serve the fish and vegetables in the parchment packets for an elegant presentation.

Nutrition Info (per serving):
- Calories: 280
- Protein: 28g
- Carbohydrates: 10g
- Dietary Fiber: 3g
- Sugars: 4g
- Fat: 14g
- Saturated Fat: 2g
- Sodium: 90mg

Serves: 4 Cooking Time: 25 minutes

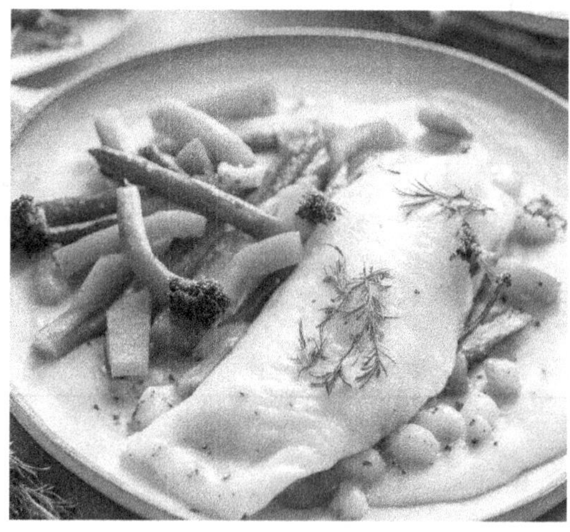

9. Salmon Berry Salad

Ingredients:

- 4 salmon fillets (about 6 ounces each)
- 2 tablespoons olive oil
- 6 cups mixed greens (spinach, arugula, kale)
- 1 cup fresh strawberries, sliced
- 1 cup fresh blueberries
- 1/4 cup sliced almonds
- 1/4 cup feta cheese, crumbled (optional)
- 1/4 cup balsamic vinegar
- 1 tablespoon honey
- 1 teaspoon Dijon mustard

Instructions:

1. Preheat the grill or oven to 375°F (190°C).
2. Brush the salmon fillets with 1 tablespoon of olive oil.
3. Grill or bake the salmon for 10-15 minutes, until cooked through and flaky. Let cool slightly and then flake into large pieces.
4. In a small bowl, whisk together the balsamic vinegar, remaining olive oil, honey, and Dijon mustard.
5. In a large bowl, combine the mixed greens, strawberries, blueberries, and almonds.
6. Drizzle the salad with the balsamic dressing and toss to combine.
7. Divide the salad among four plates and top with flaked salmon and feta cheese (if using).
8. Serve immediately.

Nutrition Info (per serving):

- Calories: 450
- Protein: 34g
- Carbohydrates: 18g
- Dietary Fiber: 5g
- Sugars: 10g
- Fat: 28g
- Saturated Fat: 5g
- Sodium: 180mg

Serves: 4 Cooking Time: 20 minutes

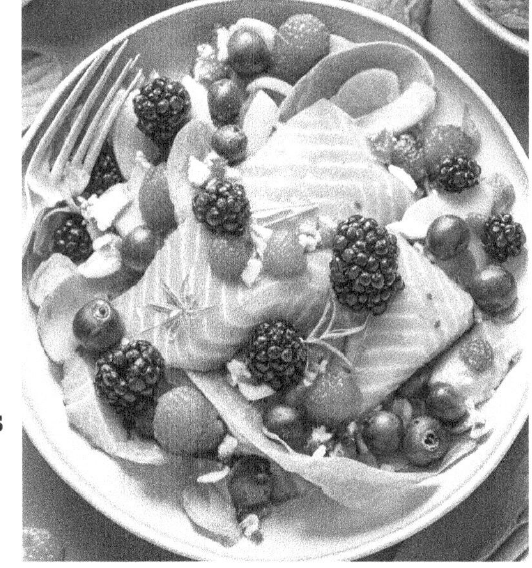

10. Sole Meuniere

Ingredients:

- 4 sole fillets (about 6 ounces each)
- 1/2 cup whole wheat flour
- 3 tablespoons olive oil
- 3 tablespoons unsalted butter
- 1 lemon, juiced
- 2 tablespoons fresh parsley, chopped

Instructions:

1. Dredge the sole fillets in the whole wheat flour, shaking off any excess.
2. Heat 2 tablespoons of olive oil and 2 tablespoons of butter in a large skillet over medium-high heat.
3. Add the sole fillets to the skillet and cook for 2-3 minutes on each side, until golden brown and cooked through. Transfer to a plate and keep warm.
4. Add the remaining tablespoon of butter to the skillet. Once melted, stir in the lemon juice and cook for 1 minute.
5. Pour the lemon-butter sauce over the sole fillets.
6. Sprinkle with fresh parsley and serve immediately.

Nutrition Info (per serving):

- Calories: 350
- Protein: 28g
- Carbohydrates: 10g
- Dietary Fiber: 1g
- Sugars: 1g
- Fat: 22g
- Saturated Fat: 8g
- Sodium: 90mg

Serves: 4 Cooking Time: 15 minutes

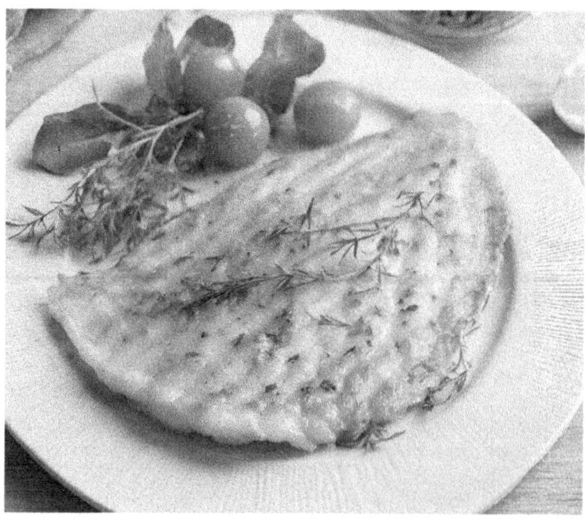

11. Asian-Style Steamed Snapper

Ingredients:

- 4 snapper fillets (about 6 ounces each)
- 2 tablespoons soy sauce (low sodium)
- 1 tablespoon rice vinegar
- 1 tablespoon sesame oil
- 1 teaspoon grated fresh ginger
- 2 garlic cloves, minced
- 2 green onions, sliced
- 1 red chili, thinly sliced (optional)
- 1/4 cup fresh cilantro, chopped

Instructions:

1. In a small bowl, combine the soy sauce, rice vinegar, sesame oil, grated ginger, and minced garlic.
2. Place each snapper fillet on a piece of parchment paper or aluminum foil.
3. Drizzle the soy sauce mixture evenly over each fillet.
4. Top with sliced green onions and red chili (if using).
5. Fold the parchment or foil around the fish to make a sealed packet.
6. Steam the fish packets in a steamer or over boiling water for 10-12 minutes, until the fish is cooked through and flakes easily with a fork.
7. Carefully open the packets and transfer the fish to plates.
8. Sprinkle with fresh cilantro and serve immediately.

Nutrition Info (per serving):

- Calories: 250
- Protein: 34g
- Carbohydrates: 3g
- Dietary Fiber: 1g
- Sugars: 1g
- Fat: 10g
- Saturated Fat: 2g
- Sodium: 300mg

Serves: 4 Cooking Time: 20 minutes

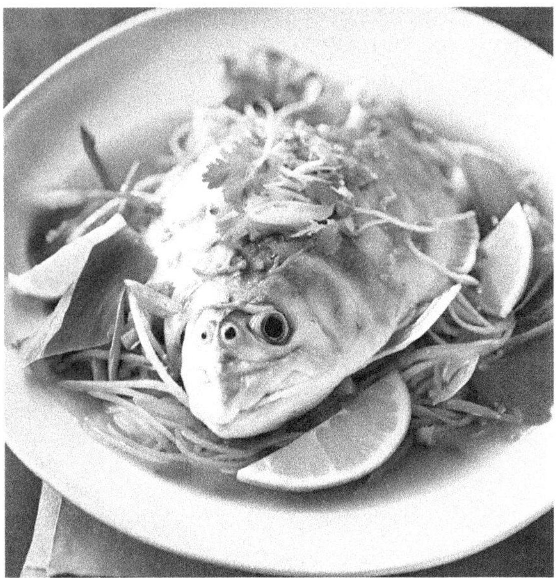

12. Peppered Mackerel with Horseradish Cream

Ingredients:

- 4 mackerel fillets (about 6 ounces each)
- 2 tablespoons olive oil
- 2 teaspoons coarsely ground black pepper
- 1/2 cup Greek yogurt
- 1 tablespoon prepared horseradish
- 1 tablespoon lemon juice
- 1 tablespoon fresh dill, chopped

Instructions:

1. Preheat the oven to 400°F (200°C). Line a baking sheet with parchment paper.
2. Rub the mackerel fillets with olive oil and coat with coarsely ground black pepper.
3. Place the mackerel fillets on the prepared baking sheet and bake for 12-15 minutes, until the fish is cooked through and flakes easily with a fork.
4. In a small bowl, mix the Greek yogurt, prepared horseradish, lemon juice, and chopped dill to make the horseradish cream.
5. Serve the baked mackerel fillets topped with the horseradish cream.

Nutrition Info (per serving):

- Calories: 350
- Protein: 28g
- Carbohydrates: 3g
- Dietary Fiber: 1g
- Sugars: 2g
- Fat: 24g
- Saturated Fat: 6g
- Sodium: 150mg

Serves: 4 Cooking Time: 20 minutes

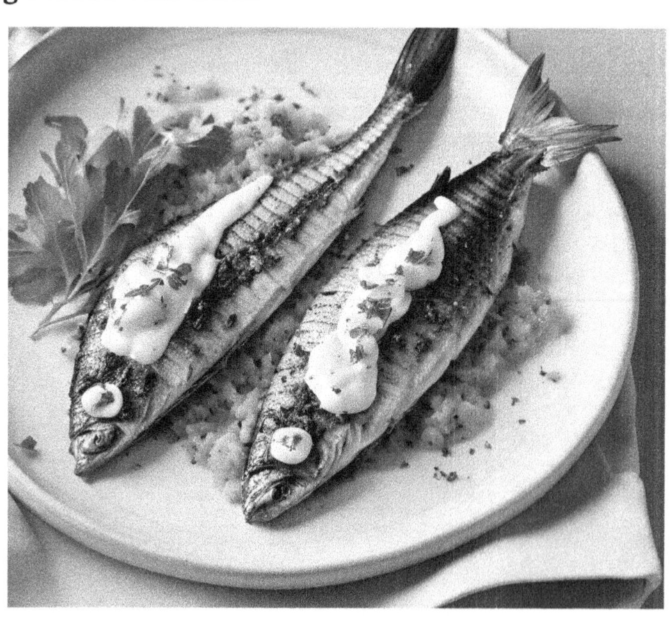

13. Baked Trout with Herb Butter

Ingredients:

- 4 trout fillets (about 6 ounces each)
- 1/4 cup unsalted butter, softened
- 2 tablespoons fresh parsley, chopped
- 1 tablespoon fresh chives, chopped
- 1 tablespoon fresh tarragon, chopped
- 1 lemon, thinly sliced

Instructions:

1. Preheat the oven to 375°F (190°C). Line a baking sheet with parchment paper.
2. In a small bowl, mix the softened butter with the parsley, chives, and tarragon.
3. Place the trout fillets on the prepared baking sheet.
4. Spread the herb butter evenly over each fillet.
5. Arrange lemon slices on top of the trout fillets.
6. Bake for 15-20 minutes, until the trout is cooked through and flakes easily with a fork.
7. Serve immediately.

Nutrition Info (per serving):

- Calories: 320
- Protein: 28g
- Carbohydrates: 2g
- Dietary Fiber: 1g
- Sugars: 0g
- Fat: 22g
- Saturated Fat: 10g
- Sodium: 90mg

Serves: 4 Cooking Time: 20 minutes

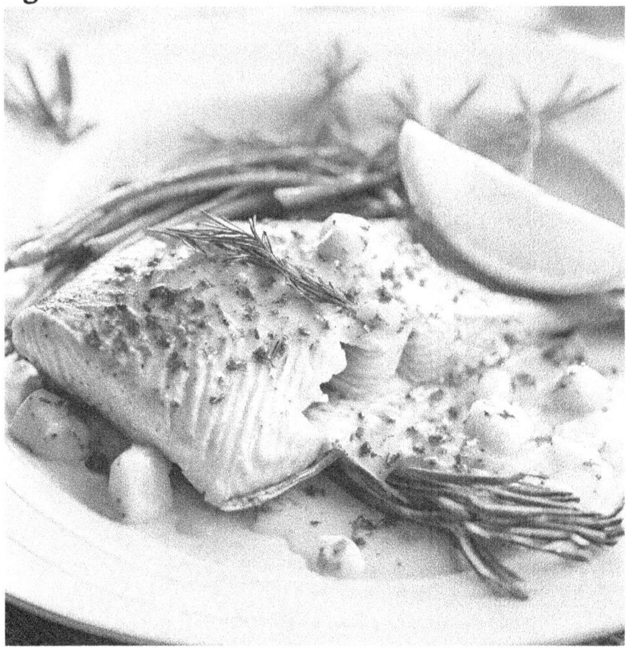

14. Lemon Garlic Tilapia

Ingredients:

- 4 tilapia fillets (about 6 ounces each)
- 3 tablespoons olive oil
- 3 garlic cloves, minced
- 1 lemon, juiced and zested
- 1 tablespoon fresh parsley, chopped
- 1/4 teaspoon paprika

Instructions:

1. Preheat the oven to 375°F (190°C). Line a baking sheet with parchment paper.
2. In a small bowl, mix the olive oil, minced garlic, lemon juice, lemon zest, and paprika.
3. Place the tilapia fillets on the prepared baking sheet.
4. Brush the olive oil mixture evenly over the fillets.
5. Bake for 15-20 minutes, until the fish is cooked through and flakes easily with a fork.
6. Garnish with chopped parsley and serve immediately.

Nutrition Info (per serving):

- Calories: 280
- Protein: 32g
- Carbohydrates: 3g
- Dietary Fiber: 0g
- Sugars: 0g
- Fat: 16g
- Saturated Fat: 2.5g
- Sodium: 70mg

Serves: 4 Cooking Time: 20 minutes

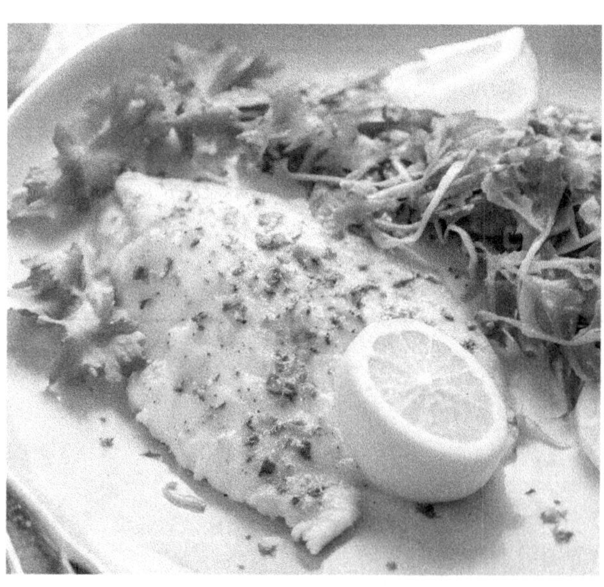

15. Moroccan Spiced Salmon

Ingredients:

- 4 salmon fillets (about 6 ounces each)
- 2 tablespoons olive oil
- 1 teaspoon ground cumin
- 1 teaspoon ground coriander
- 1 teaspoon paprika
- 1/2 teaspoon ground cinnamon
- 1/4 teaspoon ground turmeric
- 1 lemon, sliced

Instructions:

1. Preheat the oven to 375°F (190°C). Line a baking sheet with parchment paper.
2. In a small bowl, mix the olive oil, ground cumin, ground coriander, paprika, ground cinnamon, and ground turmeric.
3. Rub the spice mixture evenly over the salmon fillets.
4. Place the salmon fillets on the prepared baking sheet and top with lemon slices.
5. Bake for 15-20 minutes, until the salmon is cooked through and flakes easily with a fork.
6. Serve immediately.

Nutrition Info (per serving):

- Calories: 360
- Protein: 34g
- Carbohydrates: 2g
- Dietary Fiber: 1g
- Sugars: 0g
- Fat: 22g
- Saturated Fat: 4g
- Sodium: 60mg

Serves: 4 Cooking Time: 20 minutes

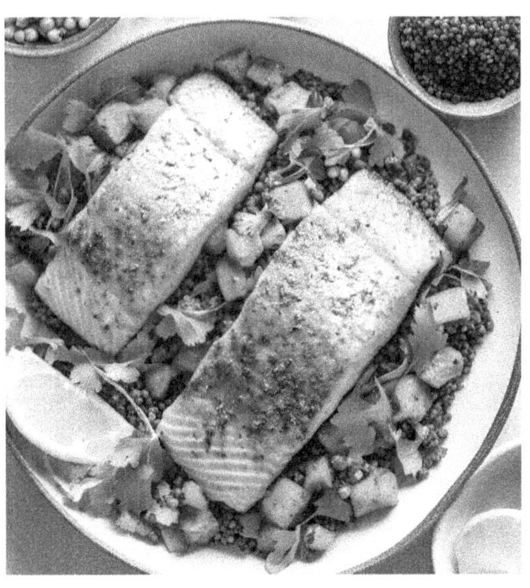

16. Shrimp Gazpacho

Ingredients:

- 1 pound large shrimp, peeled and deveined
- 4 cups tomato juice (low sodium)
- 1 cucumber, peeled and diced
- 1 red bell pepper, diced
- 1 green bell pepper, diced
- 1 small red onion, finely chopped
- 2 garlic cloves, minced
- 1/4 cup red wine vinegar
- 2 tablespoons olive oil
- 1 teaspoon smoked paprika
- 1/4 cup fresh cilantro, chopped
- 1 avocado, diced (optional)

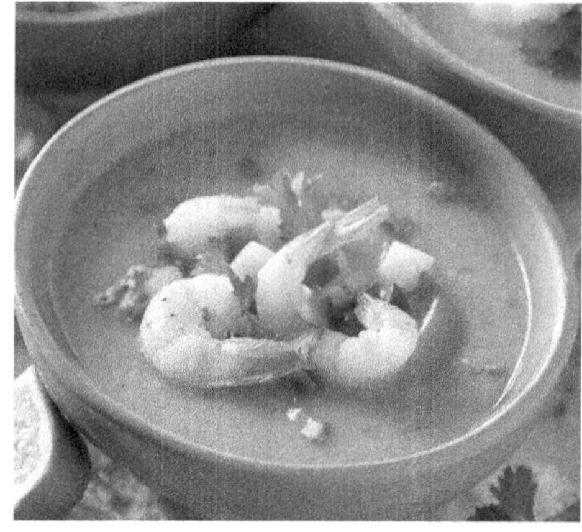

Instructions:

1. In a large pot, bring water to a boil. Add the shrimp and cook for 2-3 minutes until pink and opaque. Drain and let cool, then chop into bite-sized pieces.
2. In a large bowl, combine the tomato juice, cucumber, red bell pepper, green bell pepper, red onion, minced garlic, red wine vinegar, olive oil, and smoked paprika.
3. Add the chopped shrimp and mix well.
4. Cover and refrigerate for at least 2 hours to allow the flavors to meld.
5. Serve chilled, garnished with fresh cilantro and diced avocado if desired.

Nutrition Info (per serving):

- Calories: 220
- Protein: 20g
- Carbohydrates: 15g
- Dietary Fiber: 4g
- Sugars: 10g
- Fat: 10g
- Saturated Fat: 1.5g
- Sodium: 320mg

Serves: 4 Cooking Time: 10 minutes (plus 2 hours chilling time)

17. Sea Bass with Fennel and Orange

Ingredients:

- 4 sea bass fillets (about 6 ounces each)
- 2 tablespoons olive oil
- 1 fennel bulb, thinly sliced
- 1 orange, thinly sliced
- 1 tablespoon fresh thyme leaves
- 1/4 teaspoon ground cumin

Instructions:

1. Preheat the oven to 375°F (190°C). Line a baking sheet with parchment paper.
2. Arrange the fennel slices and orange slices on the baking sheet.
3. Place the sea bass fillets on top of the fennel and orange slices.
4. Drizzle with olive oil and sprinkle with fresh thyme leaves and ground cumin.
5. Bake for 20-25 minutes, until the sea bass is cooked through and flakes easily with a fork.
6. Serve immediately.

Nutrition Info (per serving):

- Calories: 310
- Protein: 30g
- Carbohydrates: 8g
- Dietary Fiber: 3g
- Sugars: 4g
- Fat: 18g
- Saturated Fat: 3g
- Sodium: 90mg

Serves: 4 Cooking Time: 25 minutes

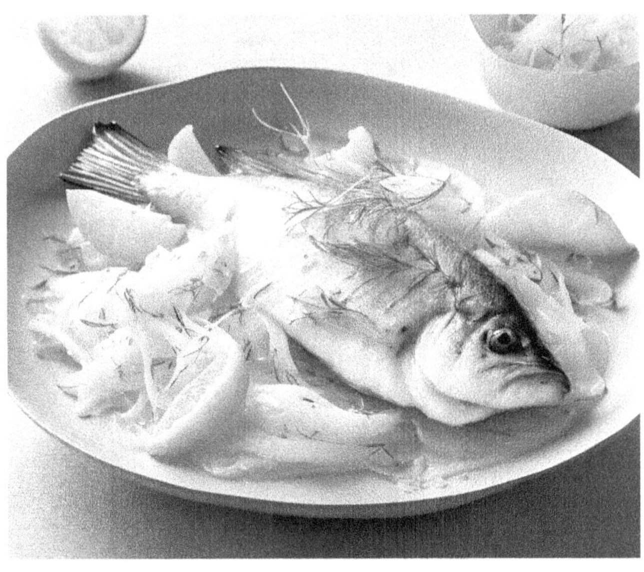

18. Cod with Parsley Pesto

Ingredients:

- 4 cod fillets (about 6 ounces each)
- 1 cup fresh parsley leaves
- 1/4 cup walnuts
- 2 garlic cloves
- 1/4 cup olive oil
- 1 lemon, juiced and zested

Instructions:

1. Preheat the oven to 375°F (190°C). Line a baking sheet with parchment paper.
2. In a food processor, combine the parsley leaves, walnuts, garlic cloves, olive oil, lemon juice, and lemon zest. Blend until smooth to make the pesto.
3. Place the cod fillets on the prepared baking sheet.
4. Spread the parsley pesto evenly over each fillet.
5. Bake for 15-20 minutes, until the cod is cooked through and flakes easily with a fork.
6. Serve immediately.

Nutrition Info (per serving):

- Calories: 330
- Protein: 34g
- Carbohydrates: 4g
- Dietary Fiber: 1g
- Sugars: 0g
- Fat: 20g
- Saturated Fat: 3g
- Sodium: 90mg

Serves: 4 Cooking Time: 20 minutes

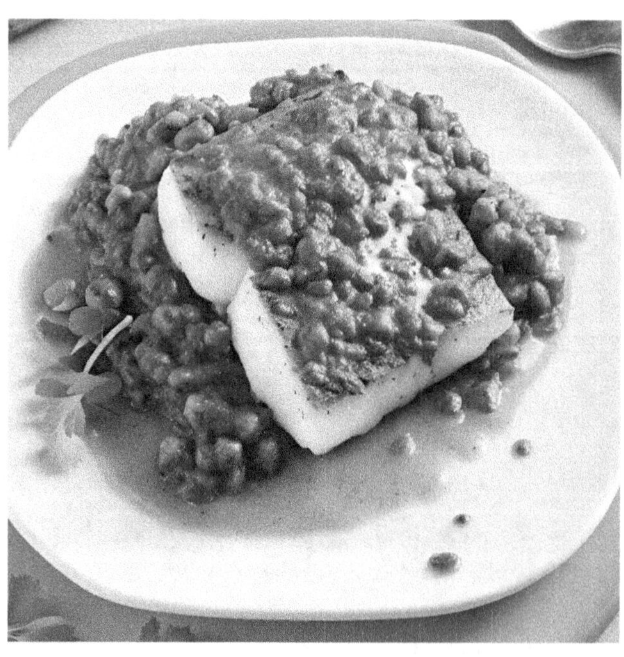

19. Salmon Quiche with Dill

Ingredients:

- 1 pre-made whole wheat pie crust
- 6 ounces cooked salmon, flaked
- 1 cup fresh spinach, chopped
- 1/2 cup feta cheese, crumbled
- 4 large eggs
- 1 cup unsweetened almond milk
- 1/4 cup fresh dill, chopped
- 1/2 teaspoon garlic powder
- 1/2 teaspoon paprika

Instructions:

1. Preheat the oven to 375°F (190°C).
2. Place the pre-made pie crust in a 9-inch pie dish.
3. Spread the flaked salmon evenly over the bottom of the pie crust.
4. Add the chopped spinach and feta cheese on top of the salmon.
5. In a medium bowl, whisk together the eggs, almond milk, dill, garlic powder, and paprika.
6. Pour the egg mixture over the salmon, spinach, and feta in the pie crust.
7. Bake for 35-40 minutes, until the quiche is set and golden brown on top.
8. Allow the quiche to cool slightly before slicing and serving.

Nutrition Info (per serving):

- Calories: 250
- Protein: 16g
- Carbohydrates: 16g
- Dietary Fiber: 2g
- Sugars: 2g
- Fat: 14g
- Saturated Fat: 4g
- Sodium: 300mg

Serves: 6 Cooking Time: 45 minutes

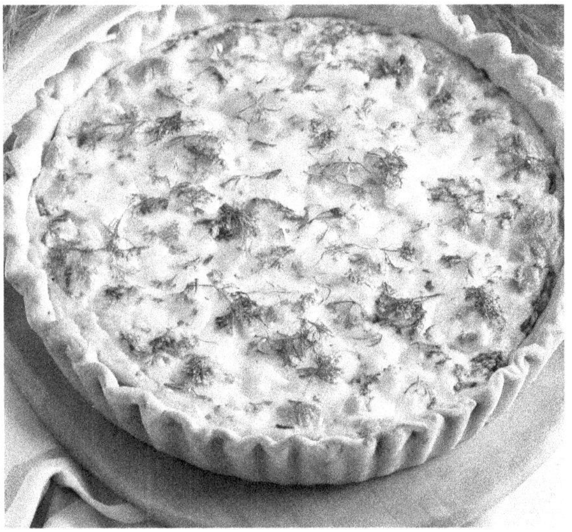

20. Prawn Stir-Fry with Bell Peppers

Ingredients:

- 1 pound large prawns, peeled and deveined
- 2 tablespoons olive oil
- 1 red bell pepper, thinly sliced
- 1 yellow bell pepper, thinly sliced
- 1 green bell pepper, thinly sliced
- 2 garlic cloves, minced
- 1 tablespoon ginger, minced
- 2 tablespoons low-sodium soy sauce
- 1 tablespoon rice vinegar
- 1 teaspoon sesame oil
- 1 tablespoon sesame seeds
- 1/4 cup fresh cilantro, chopped

Instructions:

1. Heat the olive oil in a large skillet or wok over medium-high heat.
2. Add the minced garlic and ginger, and stir-fry for about 1 minute until fragrant.
3. Add the sliced bell peppers and stir-fry for 3-4 minutes until they start to soften.
4. Add the prawns to the skillet and cook for 3-4 minutes until they turn pink and opaque.
5. Stir in the soy sauce, rice vinegar, and sesame oil. Cook for another 1-2 minutes until everything is well coated and heated through.
6. Sprinkle with sesame seeds and fresh cilantro before serving.

Nutrition Info (per serving):

- Calories: 240
- Protein: 24g
- Carbohydrates: 10g
- Dietary Fiber: 3g
- Sugars: 4g
- Fat: 12g
- Saturated Fat: 2g
- Sodium: 450mg

Serves: 4 Cooking Time: 15 minutes

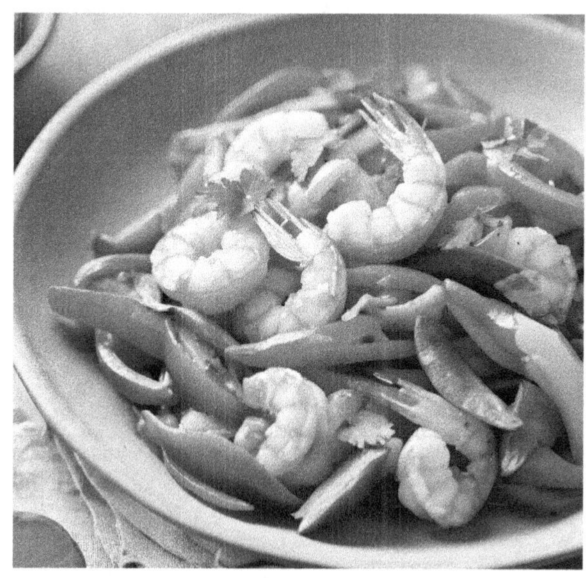

21. Tilapia with Mango Salsa

Ingredients:

- 4 tilapia fillets (about 6 ounces each)
- 2 tablespoons olive oil
- 1 teaspoon ground cumin
- 1 teaspoon paprika
- 1 large mango, peeled and diced
- 1/2 red onion, finely chopped
- 1/2 red bell pepper, diced
- 1/4 cup fresh cilantro, chopped
- 1 lime, juiced

Instructions:

1. Preheat the oven to 375°F (190°C). Line a baking sheet with parchment paper.
2. In a small bowl, mix the olive oil, ground cumin, and paprika.
3. Brush the tilapia fillets with the olive oil mixture.
4. Place the tilapia fillets on the prepared baking sheet and bake for 15-20 minutes, until the fish is cooked through and flakes easily with a fork.
5. While the fish is baking, prepare the mango salsa. In a medium bowl, combine the diced mango, red onion, red bell pepper, cilantro, and lime juice.
6. Serve the baked tilapia topped with the fresh mango salsa.

Nutrition Info (per serving):

- Calories: 280
- Protein: 28g
- Carbohydrates: 14g
- Dietary Fiber: 2g
- Sugars: 10g
- Fat: 14g
- Saturated Fat: 2g
- Sodium: 90mg

Serves: 4 Cooking Time: 20 minutes

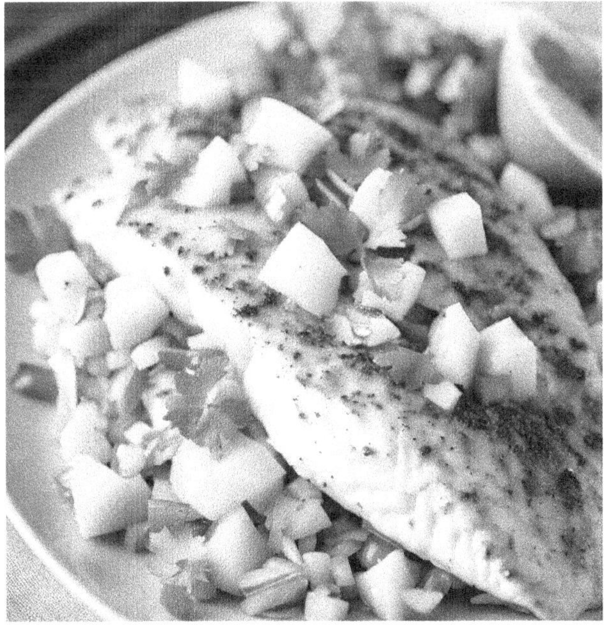

22. Flounder Piccata
Ingredients:
- 4 flounder fillets (about 6 ounces each)
- 1/2 cup whole wheat flour
- 2 tablespoons olive oil
- 1/4 cup lemon juice
- 1/4 cup vegetable broth (low sodium)
- 2 tablespoons capers, rinsed and drained
- 1/4 cup fresh parsley, chopped
- 1 lemon, sliced for garnish

Instructions:
1. Dredge the flounder fillets in whole wheat flour, shaking off any excess.
2. Heat the olive oil in a large skillet over medium-high heat.
3. Add the flounder fillets and cook for 2-3 minutes on each side, until golden brown and cooked through. Remove the fillets and set aside.
4. In the same skillet, add lemon juice, vegetable broth, and capers. Bring to a boil, scraping up any browned bits from the bottom of the skillet.
5. Reduce the heat and simmer for 2 minutes until the sauce thickens slightly.
6. Return the flounder fillets to the skillet and coat them with the sauce.
7. Garnish with chopped parsley and lemon slices. Serve immediately.

Nutrition Info (per serving):
- Calories: 250
- Protein: 28g
- Carbohydrates: 10g
- Dietary Fiber: 2g
- Sugars: 1g
- Fat: 10g
- Saturated Fat: 1.5g
- Sodium: 220mg

Serves: 4 Cooking Time: 15 minutes

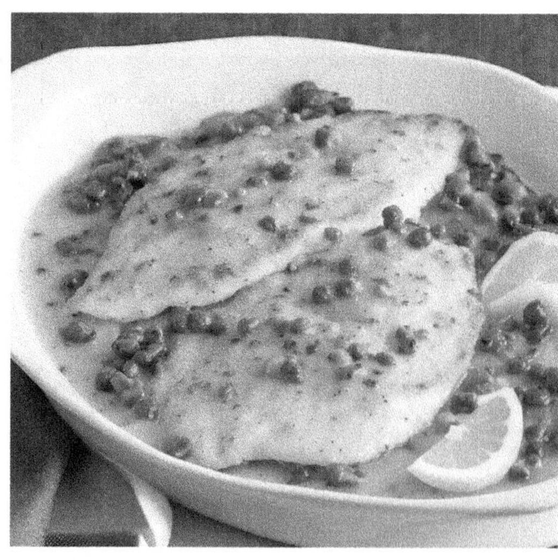

23. Halibut with Tomato Caper Sauce

Ingredients:

- 4 halibut fillets (about 6 ounces each)
- 2 tablespoons olive oil
- 1 medium onion, finely chopped
- 3 garlic cloves, minced
- 1 can (14.5 ounces) diced tomatoes, with juice
- 2 tablespoons capers, rinsed and drained
- 1 teaspoon dried oregano
- 1/4 cup fresh basil, chopped

Instructions:

1. Preheat the oven to 375°F (190°C). Line a baking dish with parchment paper.
2. Heat 1 tablespoon of olive oil in a large skillet over medium heat.
3. Add the chopped onion and cook until softened, about 5 minutes.
4. Add the minced garlic and cook for another minute.
5. Stir in the diced tomatoes, capers, and dried oregano. Simmer for 10 minutes, until the sauce thickens slightly.
6. Place the halibut fillets in the prepared baking dish and spoon the tomato caper sauce over the top.
7. Bake for 15-20 minutes, until the halibut is cooked through and flakes easily with a fork.
8. Garnish with fresh basil and serve immediately.

Nutrition Info (per serving):

- Calories: 280
- Protein: 32g
- Carbohydrates: 8g
- Dietary Fiber: 2g
- Sugars: 4g
- Fat: 12g
- Saturated Fat: 2g
- Sodium: 300mg

Serves: 4 Cooking Time: 30 minutes

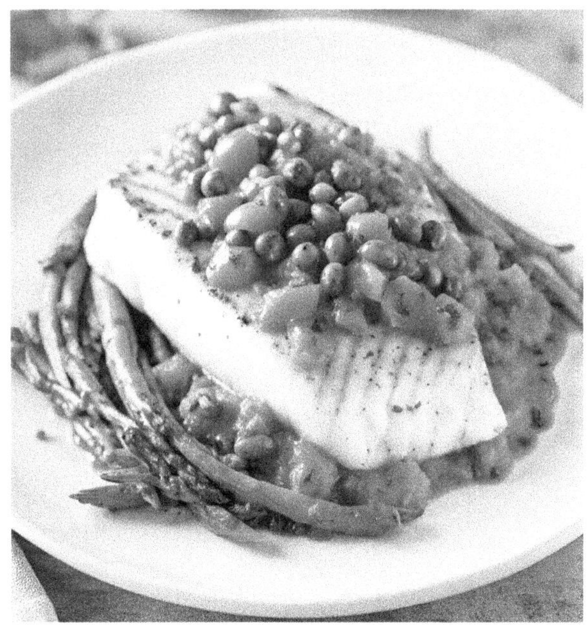

24. Miso-Glazed Cod

Ingredients:

- 4 cod fillets (about 6 ounces each)
- 2 tablespoons miso paste
- 1 tablespoon rice vinegar
- 1 tablespoon mirin
- 1 tablespoon soy sauce (low sodium)
- 1 teaspoon grated fresh ginger
- 1 garlic clove, minced

Instructions:

1. Preheat the oven to 400°F (200°C). Line a baking sheet with parchment paper.
2. In a small bowl, mix the miso paste, rice vinegar, mirin, soy sauce, grated ginger, and minced garlic until smooth.
3. Brush the miso glaze evenly over the cod fillets.
4. Place the cod fillets on the prepared baking sheet and bake for 15-20 minutes, until the fish is cooked through and flakes easily with a fork.
5. Serve immediately.

Nutrition Info (per serving):

- Calories: 210
- Protein: 32g
- Carbohydrates: 4g
- Dietary Fiber: 0g
- Sugars: 2g
- Fat: 6g
- Saturated Fat: 1g
- Sodium: 400mg

Serves: 4 Cooking Time: 20 minutes

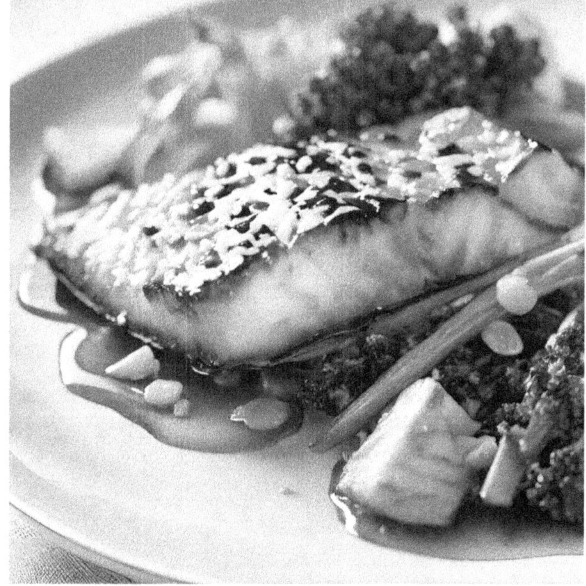

25. Lemon Baked Perch

Ingredients:

- 4 perch fillets (about 6 ounces each)
- 2 tablespoons olive oil
- 2 garlic cloves, minced
- 1 lemon, thinly sliced
- 1 tablespoon fresh thyme leaves
- 1/4 cup fresh parsley, chopped

Instructions:

1. Preheat the oven to 375°F (190°C). Line a baking sheet with parchment paper.
2. In a small bowl, mix the olive oil and minced garlic.
3. Place the perch fillets on the prepared baking sheet.
4. Brush the olive oil mixture evenly over the fillets.
5. Arrange lemon slices on top of the perch fillets and sprinkle with fresh thyme leaves.
6. Bake for 15-20 minutes, until the fish is cooked through and flakes easily with a fork.
7. Garnish with chopped parsley and serve immediately.

Nutrition Info (per serving):

- Calories: 220
- Protein: 28g
- Carbohydrates: 3g
- Dietary Fiber: 1g
- Sugars: 0g
- Fat: 11g
- Saturated Fat: 1.5g
- Sodium: 80mg

Serves: 4 Cooking Time: 20 minutes

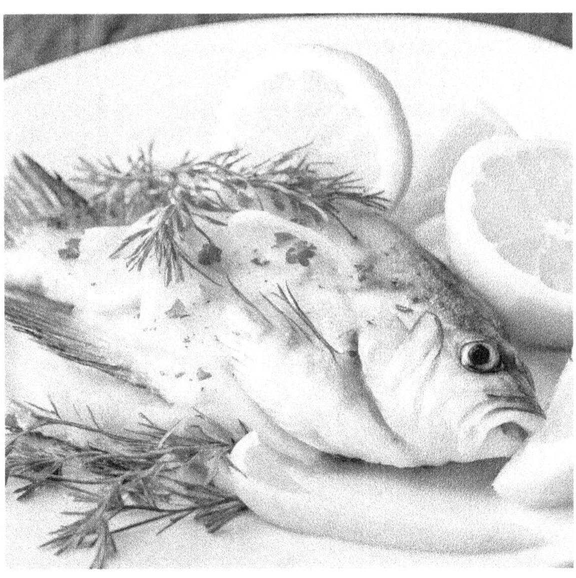

26. Ginger Soy Marinated Tuna

Ingredients:

- 4 tuna steaks (about 6 ounces each)
- 1/4 cup soy sauce (low sodium)
- 2 tablespoons rice vinegar
- 1 tablespoon honey
- 1 tablespoon grated fresh ginger
- 2 garlic cloves, minced
- 1 tablespoon sesame oil
- 2 green onions, sliced
- 1 tablespoon sesame seeds

Instructions:

1. In a bowl, mix the soy sauce, rice vinegar, honey, grated ginger, minced garlic, and sesame oil.
2. Place the tuna steaks in a shallow dish and pour the marinade over them. Cover and refrigerate for at least 30 minutes, turning the steaks occasionally.
3. Preheat the grill to medium-high heat.
4. Remove the tuna steaks from the marinade and grill for about 3-4 minutes per side, or until desired doneness.
5. Garnish with sliced green onions and sesame seeds before serving.

Nutrition Info (per serving):

- Calories: 290
- Protein: 35g
- Carbohydrates: 6g
- Dietary Fiber: 1g
- Sugars: 4g
- Fat: 14g
- Saturated Fat: 2g
- Sodium: 520mg

Serves: 4 Cooking Time: 15 minutes (plus 30 minutes marinating time)

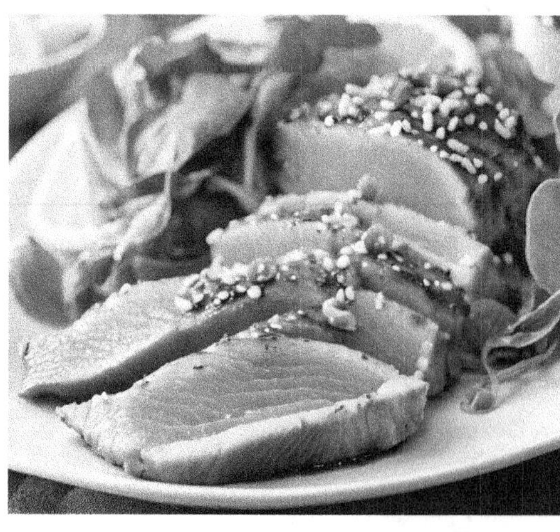

27. Pistachio-Crusted Salmon

Ingredients:

- 4 salmon fillets (about 6 ounces each)
- 1/2 cup shelled pistachios, finely chopped
- 2 tablespoons whole wheat breadcrumbs
- 2 tablespoons fresh parsley, chopped
- 2 tablespoons olive oil
- 1 lemon, zested and juiced
- 2 garlic cloves, minced

Instructions:

1. Preheat the oven to 375°F (190°C). Line a baking sheet with parchment paper.
2. In a bowl, mix the chopped pistachios, whole wheat breadcrumbs, parsley, lemon zest, and minced garlic.
3. Brush the salmon fillets with olive oil.
4. Press the pistachio mixture onto the top of each salmon fillet.
5. Place the fillets on the prepared baking sheet and bake for 15-20 minutes, until the salmon is cooked through and flakes easily with a fork.
6. Drizzle with lemon juice before serving.

Nutrition Info (per serving):

- Calories: 420
- Protein: 34g
- Carbohydrates: 8g
- Dietary Fiber: 3g
- Sugars: 1g
- Fat: 28g
- Saturated Fat: 4g
- Sodium: 110mg

Serves: 4 Cooking Time: 20 minutes

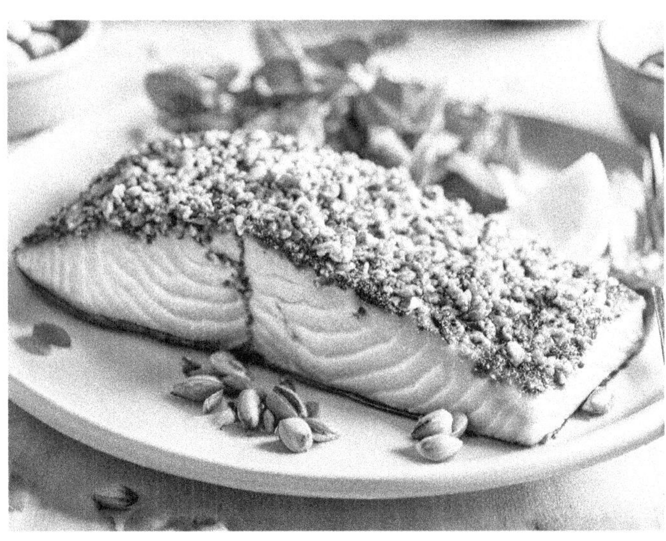

28. Anchovy Pasta with Garlic and Olive Oil

Ingredients:

- 8 ounces whole wheat spaghetti
- 1/4 cup extra-virgin olive oil
- 6 anchovy fillets, minced
- 4 garlic cloves, thinly sliced
- 1/4 teaspoon red pepper flakes (optional)
- 1/4 cup fresh parsley, chopped
- 1 lemon, zested and juiced

Instructions:

1. Cook the whole wheat spaghetti according to package instructions until al dente. Drain and set aside.
2. In a large skillet, heat the olive oil over medium heat.
3. Add the minced anchovy fillets and cook, stirring, until they dissolve in the oil, about 2-3 minutes.
4. Add the sliced garlic and red pepper flakes (if using) and cook until the garlic is golden brown, about 2 minutes.
5. Add the cooked spaghetti to the skillet and toss to coat with the anchovy-garlic oil.
6. Stir in the chopped parsley, lemon zest, and lemon juice.
7. Serve immediately.

Nutrition Info (per serving):

- Calories: 400
- Protein: 16g
- Carbohydrates: 54g
- Dietary Fiber: 8g
- Sugars: 2g
- Fat: 14g
- Saturated Fat: 2g
- Sodium: 360mg

Serves: 4 Cooking Time: 20 minutes

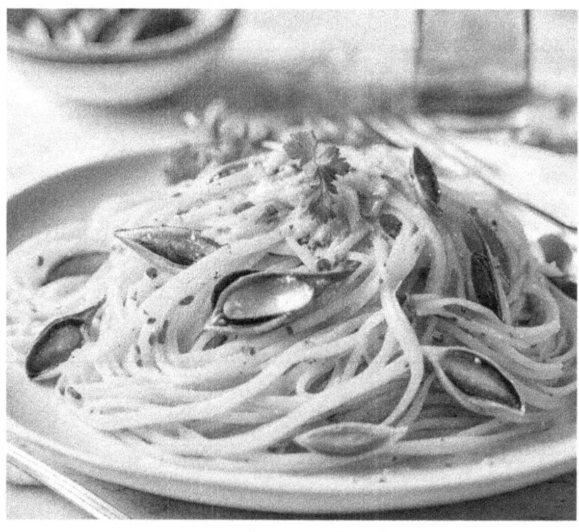

Poultry Recipes

1. Lemon Herb Roasted Chicken

Ingredients:

- 1 whole chicken (about 4 pounds)
- 1/4 cup olive oil
- 1 lemon, zested and juiced
- 4 garlic cloves, minced
- 1 tablespoon fresh rosemary, chopped
- 1 tablespoon fresh thyme, chopped
- 1 tablespoon fresh parsley, chopped
- 1/2 teaspoon paprika
- 1 lemon, cut into wedges (for roasting)
- 1 bunch of carrots, peeled and cut into large pieces
- 1 bunch of baby potatoes, halved

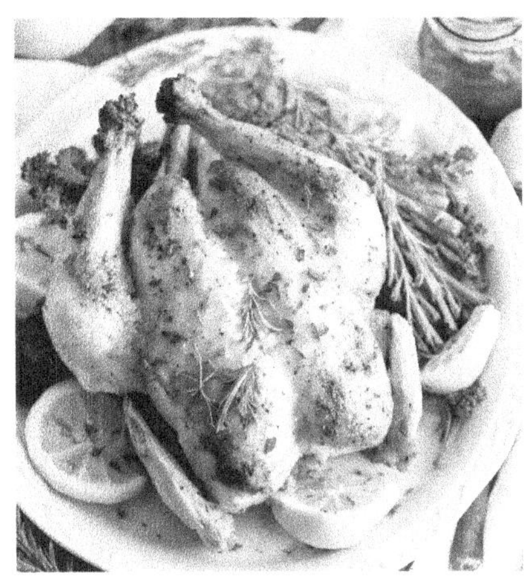

Instructions:

1. Preheat the oven to 375°F (190°C).
2. In a small bowl, mix the olive oil, lemon zest, lemon juice, minced garlic, rosemary, thyme, parsley, and paprika.
3. Place the whole chicken in a roasting pan. Rub the herb mixture all over the chicken, making sure to get some under the skin.
4. Arrange the lemon wedges, carrots, and baby potatoes around the chicken in the roasting pan.
5. Roast in the preheated oven for about 1 hour and 30 minutes, or until the internal temperature of the chicken reaches 165°F (74°C) and the vegetables are tender.
6. Let the chicken rest for 10 minutes before carving. Serve with the roasted vegetables.

Nutrition Info (per serving):

- Calories: 400
- Protein: 32g
- Carbohydrates: 20g
- Dietary Fiber: 4g
- Sugars: 3g
- Fat: 22g
- Saturated Fat: 5g
- Sodium: 110mg

Serves: 6 Cooking Time: 1 hour 30 minutes

2. Turkey and Spinach Meatballs

Ingredients:

- 1 pound ground turkey
- 1 cup fresh spinach, finely chopped
- 1/2 cup whole wheat breadcrumbs
- 1/4 cup grated Parmesan cheese
- 1 egg, beaten
- 2 garlic cloves, minced
- 1 tablespoon fresh basil, chopped
- 1 tablespoon fresh parsley, chopped
- 1 teaspoon dried oregano
- 2 tablespoons olive oil (for cooking)

Instructions:

1. Preheat the oven to 375°F (190°C). Line a baking sheet with parchment paper.
2. In a large bowl, combine the ground turkey, chopped spinach, breadcrumbs, Parmesan cheese, beaten egg, minced garlic, basil, parsley, and oregano. Mix well until all ingredients are thoroughly combined.
3. Shape the mixture into meatballs, about 1 inch in diameter, and place them on the prepared baking sheet.
4. Heat the olive oil in a large skillet over medium-high heat. Add the meatballs and cook until browned on all sides, about 5-7 minutes.
5. Transfer the browned meatballs back to the baking sheet and bake in the preheated oven for 10-15 minutes, or until the internal temperature reaches 165°F (74°C).
6. Serve the meatballs with your favorite marinara sauce or as desired.

Nutrition Info (per serving):

- Calories: 210
- Protein: 22g
- Carbohydrates: 10g
- Dietary Fiber: 2g
- Sugars: 1g
- Fat: 10g
- Saturated Fat: 2.5g
- Sodium: 250mg

Serves: 4 Cooking Time: 30 minutes

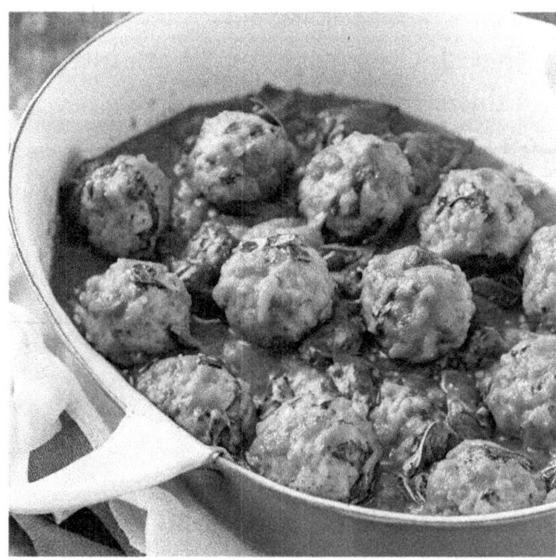

3. Chicken Ginger Soup

Ingredients:

- 1 tablespoon olive oil
- 1 medium onion, chopped
- 3 garlic cloves, minced
- 1 tablespoon fresh ginger, grated
- 1 pound boneless, skinless chicken breasts, cut into bite-sized pieces
- 6 cups low-sodium chicken broth
- 2 carrots, peeled and sliced
- 2 celery stalks, sliced
- 1 cup mushrooms, sliced
- 1 cup baby spinach
- 1 tablespoon soy sauce (low sodium)
- 1/4 cup fresh cilantro, chopped

Instructions:

1. Heat the olive oil in a large pot over medium heat.
2. Add the chopped onion and cook until softened, about 5 minutes.
3. Add the minced garlic and grated ginger, and cook for another 1-2 minutes until fragrant.
4. Add the chicken pieces to the pot and cook until no longer pink, about 5-7 minutes.
5. Pour in the chicken broth and bring to a boil.
6. Add the sliced carrots, celery, and mushrooms to the pot. Reduce the heat and simmer for 20-25 minutes, until the vegetables are tender.
7. Stir in the baby spinach and soy sauce, and cook for another 2-3 minutes until the spinach is wilted.
8. Serve the soup garnished with fresh cilantro.

Nutrition Info (per serving):

- Calories: 250
- Protein: 28g
- Carbohydrates: 14g
- Dietary Fiber: 3g
- Sugars: 5g
- Fat: 10g
- Saturated Fat: 2g
- Sodium: 300mg

Serves: 4 Cooking Time: 40 minutes

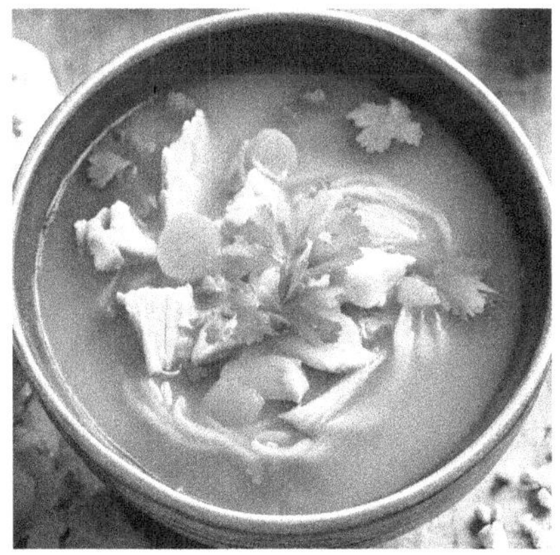

4. Baked Chicken with Prunes and Olives

Ingredients:

- 4 boneless, skinless chicken breasts
- 1/2 cup pitted prunes, chopped
- 1/2 cup green olives, pitted and sliced
- 1/4 cup olive oil
- 1/4 cup balsamic vinegar
- 1/4 cup chicken broth (low sodium)
- 2 garlic cloves, minced
- 1 teaspoon dried thyme
- 1 teaspoon paprika

Instructions:

1. Preheat the oven to 375°F (190°C). Grease a baking dish with a bit of olive oil.
2. In a bowl, mix the olive oil, balsamic vinegar, chicken broth, minced garlic, dried thyme, and paprika.
3. Place the chicken breasts in the baking dish and pour the olive oil mixture over them.
4. Scatter the chopped prunes and sliced olives around the chicken.
5. Bake for 25-30 minutes, until the chicken is cooked through and reaches an internal temperature of 165°F (74°C).
6. Serve immediately, spooning the prunes and olives over the chicken.

Nutrition Info (per serving):

- Calories: 320
- Protein: 28g
- Carbohydrates: 14g
- Dietary Fiber: 3g
- Sugars: 10g
- Fat: 18g
- Saturated Fat: 2.5g
- Sodium: 340mg

Serves: 4 Cooking Time: 30 minutes

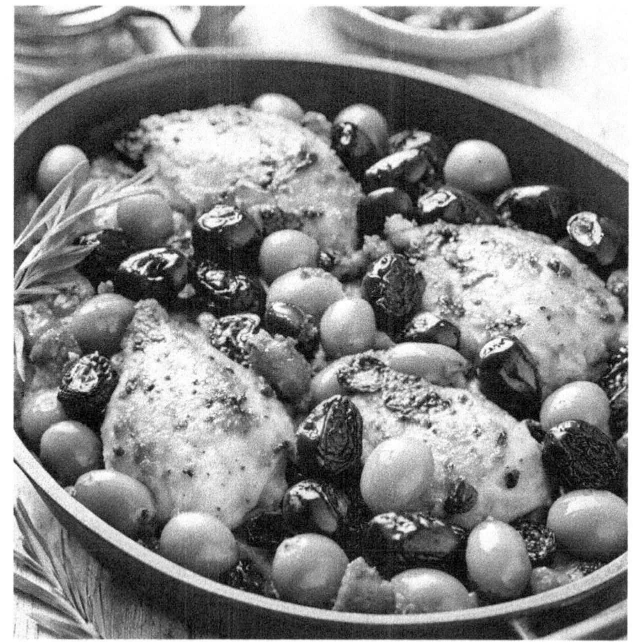

5. Grilled Turkey Burgers

Ingredients:

- 1 pound ground turkey
- 1/4 cup whole wheat breadcrumbs
- 1/4 cup grated zucchini
- 1 egg, beaten
- 2 garlic cloves, minced
- 1 tablespoon fresh parsley, chopped
- 1 tablespoon fresh basil, chopped
- 1/2 teaspoon paprika
- 1/4 teaspoon cumin
- 4 whole wheat burger buns

Instructions:

1. Preheat the grill to medium-high heat.
2. In a large bowl, mix the ground turkey, breadcrumbs, grated zucchini, beaten egg, minced garlic, parsley, basil, paprika, and cumin until well combined.
3. Shape the mixture into 4 equal-sized patties.
4. Grill the patties for about 5-7 minutes on each side, until fully cooked and the internal temperature reaches 165°F (74°C).
5. Serve the turkey burgers on whole wheat buns with your favorite toppings.

Nutrition Info (per serving):

- Calories: 320
- Protein: 28g
- Carbohydrates: 24g
- Dietary Fiber: 4g
- Sugars: 3g
- Fat: 12g
- Saturated Fat: 2g
- Sodium: 280mg

Serves: 4 Cooking Time: 15 minutes

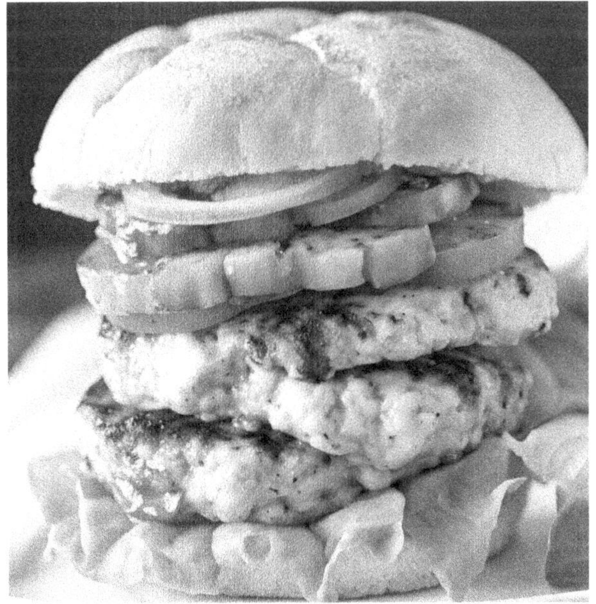

6. Chicken Salad with Avocado

Ingredients:

- 2 cups cooked chicken breast, shredded
- 1 ripe avocado, diced
- 1/2 cup cherry tomatoes, halved
- 1/2 cup cucumber, diced
- 1/4 cup red onion, finely chopped
- 1/4 cup fresh cilantro, chopped
- 2 tablespoons olive oil
- 1 lime, juiced
- 1/2 teaspoon cumin

Instructions:

1. In a large bowl, combine the shredded chicken, diced avocado, cherry tomatoes, cucumber, red onion, and fresh cilantro.
2. In a small bowl, whisk together the olive oil, lime juice, and cumin.
3. Pour the dressing over the chicken salad and toss gently to combine.
4. Serve immediately.

Nutrition Info (per serving):

- Calories: 280
- Protein: 26g
- Carbohydrates: 10g
- Dietary Fiber: 5g
- Sugars: 2g
- Fat: 16g
- Saturated Fat: 3g
- Sodium: 180mg

Serves: 4 Cooking Time: 15 minutes

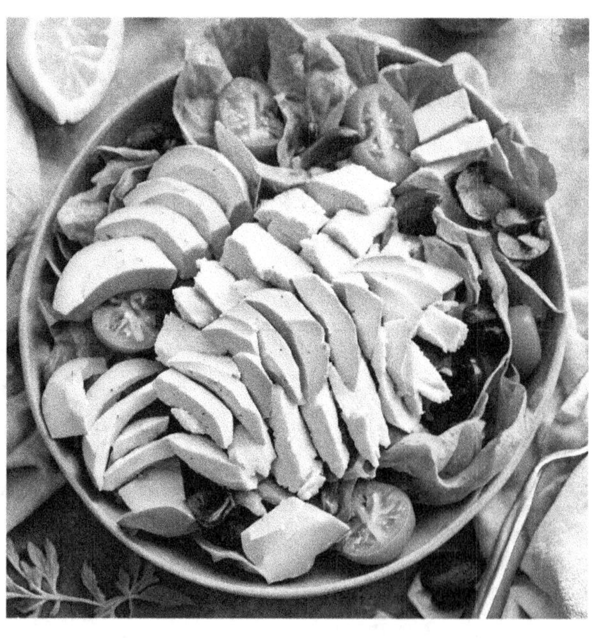

7. Turkey Chili

Ingredients:

- 1 pound ground turkey
- 1 tablespoon olive oil
- 1 large onion, chopped
- 3 garlic cloves, minced
- 1 red bell pepper, chopped
- 1 green bell pepper, chopped
- 1 can (15 ounces) kidney beans, rinsed and drained
- 1 can (15 ounces) black beans, rinsed and drained
- 1 can (14.5 ounces) diced tomatoes, with juice
- 1 cup low-sodium chicken broth
- 2 tablespoons chili powder
- 1 teaspoon ground cumin
- 1 teaspoon dried oregano

Instructions:

1. Heat the olive oil in a large pot over medium heat.
2. Add the chopped onion and minced garlic, and cook until softened, about 5 minutes.
3. Add the ground turkey and cook until browned, breaking it up with a spoon as it cooks, about 7-8 minutes.
4. Stir in the chopped red and green bell peppers, and cook for another 5 minutes.
5. Add the kidney beans, black beans, diced tomatoes, chicken broth, chili powder, ground cumin, and dried oregano. Stir to combine.
6. Bring the mixture to a boil, then reduce the heat and simmer for 30 minutes, stirring occasionally.
7. Serve hot, garnished with fresh cilantro if desired.

Nutrition Info (per serving):

- Calories: 320
- Protein: 28g
- Carbohydrates: 35g
- Dietary Fiber: 10g
- Sugars: 6g
- Fat: 10g
- Saturated Fat: 2g
- Sodium: 350mg

Serves: 6 Cooking Time: 45 minutes

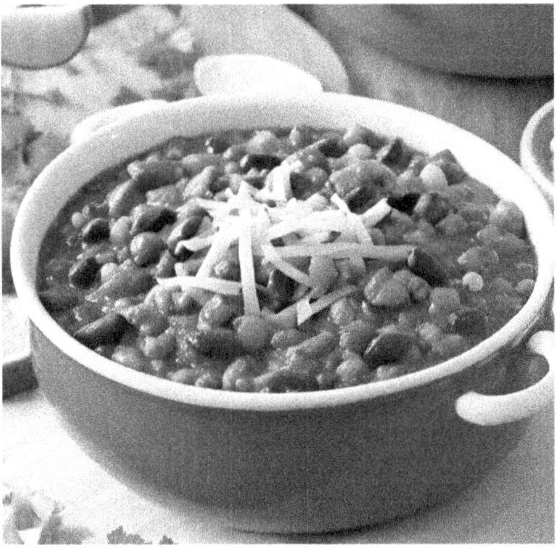

8. Poached Chicken and Vegetable Salad

Ingredients:

- 2 boneless, skinless chicken breasts
- 4 cups low-sodium chicken broth
- 1 bay leaf
- 1 cup cherry tomatoes, halved
- 1 cucumber, diced
- 1 red bell pepper, diced
- 1/2 cup red onion, finely chopped
- 4 cups mixed greens
- 1/4 cup fresh parsley, chopped
- 2 tablespoons olive oil
- 1 lemon, juiced
- 1 teaspoon Dijon mustard

Instructions:

1. In a large pot, bring the chicken broth and bay leaf to a boil.
2. Add the chicken breasts, reduce the heat, and simmer gently for 15-20 minutes, until the chicken is cooked through and reaches an internal temperature of 165°F (74°C).
3. Remove the chicken from the broth and let it cool slightly, then shred the chicken with two forks.
4. In a large bowl, combine the shredded chicken, cherry tomatoes, cucumber, red bell pepper, red onion, mixed greens, and parsley.
5. In a small bowl, whisk together the olive oil, lemon juice, and Dijon mustard.
6. Pour the dressing over the salad and toss to combine.
7. Serve immediately.

Nutrition Info (per serving):

- Calories: 220
- Protein: 24g
- Carbohydrates: 10g
- Dietary Fiber: 3g
- Sugars: 4g
- Fat: 10g
- Saturated Fat: 1.5g
- Sodium: 220mg

Serves: 4 Cooking Time: 30 minutes

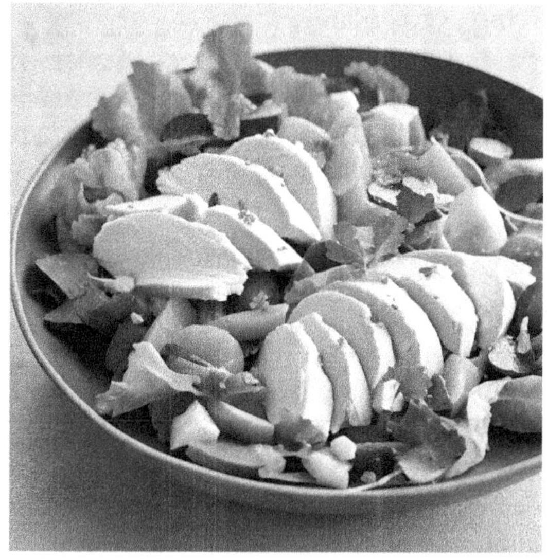

9. Chicken Cacciatore

Ingredients:

- 4 boneless, skinless chicken breasts
- 2 tablespoons olive oil
- 1 large onion, chopped
- 3 garlic cloves, minced
- 1 bell pepper, sliced
- 1 cup mushrooms, sliced
- 1 can (14.5 ounces) diced tomatoes, with juice
- 1/2 cup low-sodium chicken broth
- 1 teaspoon dried oregano
- 1 teaspoon dried basil
- 1/2 teaspoon paprika
- 1/4 cup fresh parsley, chopped

Instructions:

1. Heat the olive oil in a large skillet over medium-high heat.
2. Add the chicken breasts and cook until browned on both sides, about 5-7 minutes per side. Remove the chicken from the skillet and set aside.
3. In the same skillet, add the chopped onion and cook until softened, about 5 minutes.
4. Add the minced garlic and cook for another 1 minute.
5. Stir in the sliced bell pepper and mushrooms, and cook for 5 minutes.
6. Add the diced tomatoes, chicken broth, oregano, basil, and paprika. Stir to combine.
7. Return the chicken breasts to the skillet and bring to a simmer. Cover and cook for 20-25 minutes, until the chicken is cooked through and the sauce has thickened.
8. Garnish with chopped parsley before serving.

Nutrition Info (per serving):

- Calories: 350
- Protein: 34g
- Carbohydrates: 12g
- Dietary Fiber: 3g
- Sugars: 6g
- Fat: 18g
- Saturated Fat: 3g
- Sodium: 300mg

Serves: 4 Cooking Time: 40 minutes

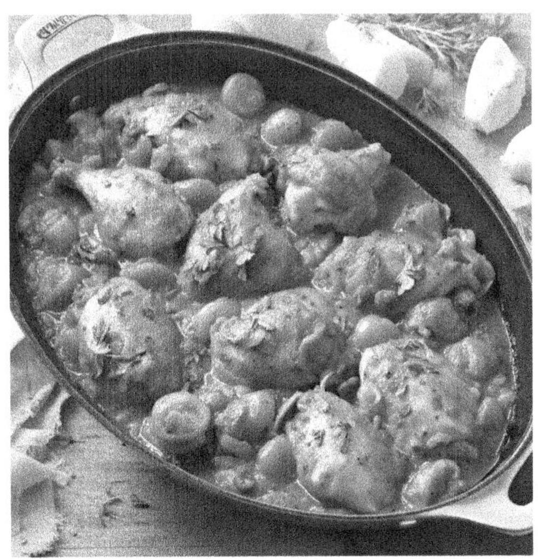

10. Stuffed Turkey Breast

Ingredients:

- 1 boneless turkey breast (about 2 pounds)
- 1 cup fresh spinach, chopped
- 1/2 cup sun-dried tomatoes, chopped
- 1/4 cup feta cheese, crumbled
- 2 garlic cloves, minced
- 2 tablespoons olive oil
- 1 teaspoon dried oregano
- 1 lemon, zested and juiced

Instructions:

1. Preheat the oven to 375°F (190°C). Grease a baking dish with a bit of olive oil.
2. In a bowl, mix the chopped spinach, sun-dried tomatoes, feta cheese, and minced garlic.
3. Butterfly the turkey breast by cutting it horizontally, being careful not to cut all the way through. Open the turkey breast like a book.
4. Spread the spinach mixture evenly over the turkey breast. Roll the turkey breast up and secure with kitchen twine.
5. In a small bowl, mix the olive oil, dried oregano, lemon zest, and lemon juice.
6. Rub the olive oil mixture all over the turkey breast.
7. Place the turkey breast in the prepared baking dish and bake for 45-50 minutes, until the internal temperature reaches 165°F (74°C).
8. Let the turkey rest for 10 minutes before slicing and serving.

Nutrition Info (per serving):

- Calories: 280
- Protein: 34g
- Carbohydrates: 6g
- Dietary Fiber: 2g
- Sugars: 2g
- Fat: 14g
- Saturated Fat: 3g
- Sodium: 320mg

Serves: 4 Cooking Time: 1 hour

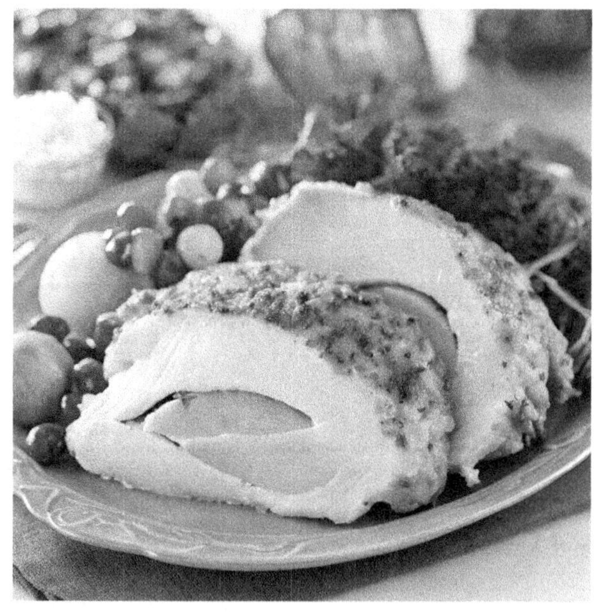

11. Roast Turkey with Citrus Glaze

Ingredients:

- 1 whole turkey (about 10 pounds)
- 1/4 cup olive oil
- 1/4 cup orange juice
- 1/4 cup lemon juice
- 1/4 cup honey
- 2 tablespoons orange zest
- 2 tablespoons lemon zest
- 3 garlic cloves, minced
- 1 tablespoon fresh thyme leaves
- 1 tablespoon fresh rosemary, chopped

Instructions:

1. Preheat the oven to 325°F (165°C). Place the turkey on a rack in a roasting pan.
2. In a small bowl, mix the olive oil, orange juice, lemon juice, honey, orange zest, lemon zest, minced garlic, thyme, and rosemary.
3. Brush the citrus glaze all over the turkey, making sure to get some under the skin.
4. Cover the turkey loosely with aluminum foil and roast in the preheated oven for 3-3.5 hours, or until the internal temperature reaches 165°F (74°C). Baste the turkey with the remaining glaze every 30 minutes.
5. Remove the foil during the last 30 minutes of roasting to allow the skin to brown.
6. Let the turkey rest for 20 minutes before carving and serving.

Nutrition Info (per serving):

- Calories: 350
- Protein: 36g
- Carbohydrates: 10g
- Dietary Fiber: 1g
- Sugars: 8g
- Fat: 18g
- Saturated Fat: 4g
- Sodium: 240mg

Serves: 8 Cooking Time: 4 hours

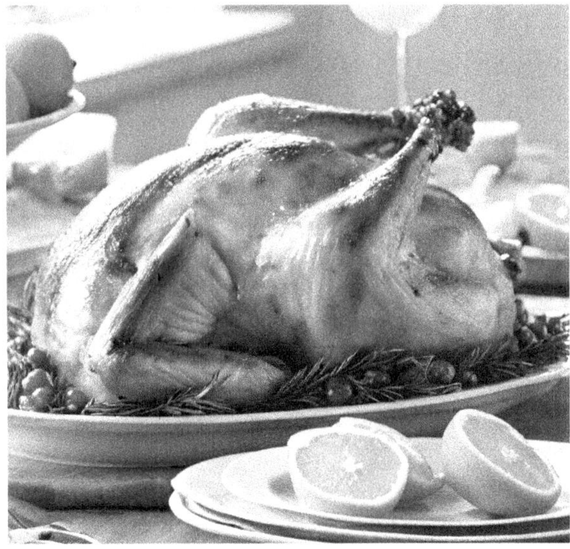

12. Chicken Pho

Ingredients:

- 8 cups low-sodium chicken broth
- 2 boneless, skinless chicken breasts
- 1 large onion, halved
- 4 garlic cloves, crushed
- 1 piece fresh ginger (2 inches), sliced
- 2 star anise
- 1 cinnamon stick
- 1 tablespoon fish sauce
- 1 tablespoon soy sauce (low sodium)
- 8 ounces rice noodles
- 1 cup bean sprouts
- 1/2 cup fresh cilantro, chopped
- 1/2 cup fresh basil leaves
- 1/2 cup fresh mint leaves
- 1 lime, cut into wedges

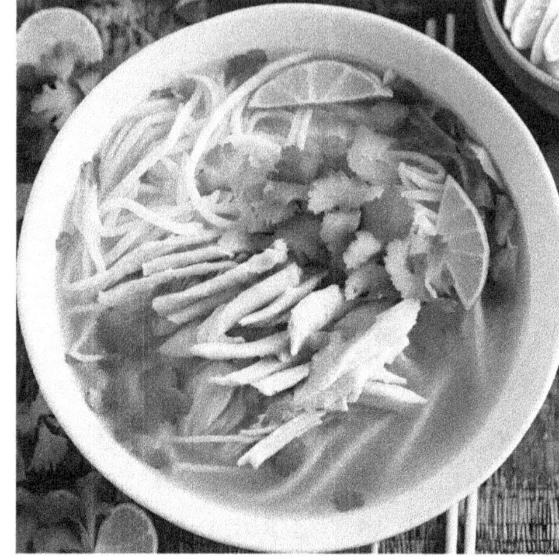

Instructions:

1. In a large pot, bring the chicken broth to a boil.
2. Add the chicken breasts, halved onion, crushed garlic, sliced ginger, star anise, and cinnamon stick to the pot. Reduce the heat and simmer for 20 minutes, until the chicken is cooked through.
3. Remove the chicken breasts from the pot and shred them with two forks. Set aside.
4. Strain the broth through a fine mesh sieve, discarding the solids, and return the broth to the pot.
5. Stir in the fish sauce and soy sauce. Keep the broth warm over low heat.
6. Cook the rice noodles according to package instructions, then drain and divide them among four bowls.
7. Top the noodles with the shredded chicken, bean sprouts, cilantro, basil, and mint.
8. Ladle the hot broth over the noodles and herbs.
9. Serve with lime wedges on the side.

Nutrition Info (per serving):

- Calories: 300
- Protein: 28g
- Carbohydrates: 35g
- Dietary Fiber: 3g
- Sugars: 3g
- Fat: 6g
- Saturated Fat: 1g
- Sodium: 400mg

Serves: 4 Cooking Time: 45 minutes

13. Moroccan Turkey Stew

Ingredients:

- 1 pound turkey breast, cut into bite-sized pieces
- 2 tablespoons olive oil
- 1 large onion, chopped
- 3 garlic cloves, minced
- 1 teaspoon ground cumin
- 1 teaspoon ground coriander
- 1 teaspoon ground cinnamon
- 1/2 teaspoon ground turmeric
- 1/2 teaspoon ground ginger
- 1 can (14.5 ounces) diced tomatoes, with juice
- 2 cups low-sodium chicken broth
- 1 cup chickpeas, cooked and drained
- 1/2 cup dried apricots, chopped
- 1/4 cup fresh cilantro, chopped

Instructions:

1. Heat the olive oil in a large pot over medium heat.
2. Add the chopped onion and cook until softened, about 5 minutes.
3. Add the minced garlic and turkey pieces, and cook until the turkey is browned on all sides, about 5-7 minutes.
4. Stir in the ground cumin, coriander, cinnamon, turmeric, and ginger. Cook for 1 minute until fragrant.
5. Add the diced tomatoes and chicken broth, and bring to a simmer.
6. Stir in the chickpeas and dried apricots.
7. Cover and simmer for 20-25 minutes, until the turkey is cooked through and the flavors have melded.
8. Garnish with fresh cilantro before serving.

Nutrition Info (per serving):

- Calories: 320
- Protein: 28g
- Carbohydrates: 28g
- Dietary Fiber: 7g
- Sugars: 12g
- Fat: 12g
- Saturated Fat: 2g
- Sodium: 350mg

Serves: 4 Cooking Time: 40 minutes

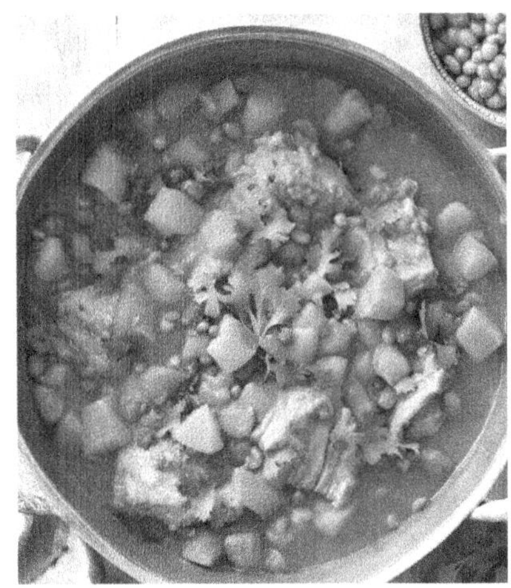

14. Turkey and Quinoa Stuffed Peppers
Ingredients:

- 4 large bell peppers
- 1 pound ground turkey
- 1 cup cooked quinoa
- 1 cup tomato sauce (low sodium)
- 1 small onion, finely chopped
- 2 garlic cloves, minced
- 1 teaspoon dried oregano
- 1 teaspoon dried basil
- 1/2 cup shredded mozzarella cheese (optional)
- 2 tablespoons olive oil

Instructions:

1. Preheat the oven to 375°F (190°C).
2. Cut the tops off the bell peppers and remove the seeds and membranes. Brush the peppers with olive oil and place them in a baking dish.
3. In a large skillet, heat the olive oil over medium heat.
4. Add the chopped onion and minced garlic, and cook until softened, about 5 minutes.
5. Add the ground turkey and cook until browned, breaking it up with a spoon, about 7-8 minutes.
6. Stir in the cooked quinoa, tomato sauce, dried oregano, and dried basil. Cook for another 5 minutes until heated through.
7. Stuff the bell peppers with the turkey and quinoa mixture.
8. If using, sprinkle the shredded mozzarella cheese on top of the stuffed peppers.
9. Cover the baking dish with foil and bake for 25 minutes.
10. Remove the foil and bake for another 10 minutes, until the peppers are tender and the cheese is melted and bubbly.
11. Serve immediately.

Nutrition Info (per serving):

- Calories: 300
- Protein: 30g
- Carbohydrates: 25g
- Dietary Fiber: 5g
- Sugars: 8g
- Fat: 10g
- Saturated Fat: 2.5g
- Sodium: 400mg

Serves: 4 Cooking Time: 45 minutes

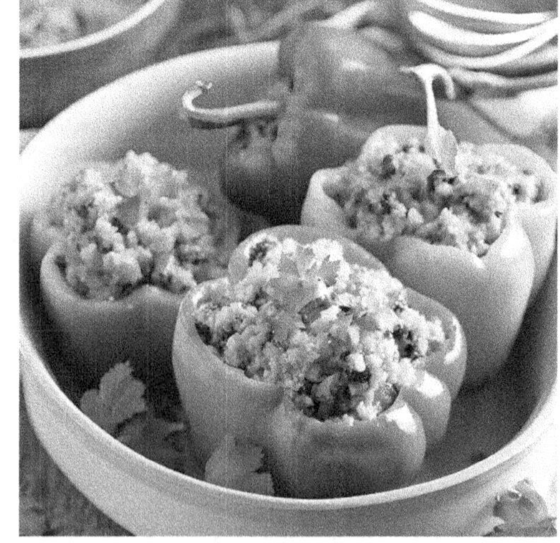

15. Turkey Piccata

Ingredients:

- 4 turkey cutlets (about 4 ounces each)
- 1/4 cup whole wheat flour
- 2 tablespoons olive oil
- 1/4 cup lemon juice
- 1/4 cup low-sodium chicken broth
- 2 tablespoons capers, rinsed and drained
- 1/4 cup fresh parsley, chopped
- 1 lemon, sliced for garnish

Instructions:

1. Dredge the turkey cutlets in whole wheat flour, shaking off any excess.
2. Heat the olive oil in a large skillet over medium-high heat.
3. Add the turkey cutlets and cook for 2-3 minutes on each side, until golden brown and cooked through. Remove the cutlets from the skillet and set aside.
4. In the same skillet, add the lemon juice, chicken broth, and capers. Bring to a boil, scraping up any browned bits from the bottom of the skillet.
5. Reduce the heat and simmer for 2 minutes until the sauce thickens slightly.
6. Return the turkey cutlets to the skillet and coat them with the sauce.
7. Garnish with chopped parsley and lemon slices. Serve immediately.

Nutrition Info (per serving):

- Calories: 260
- Protein: 28g
- Carbohydrates: 10g
- Dietary Fiber: 2g
- Sugars: 1g
- Fat: 12g
- Saturated Fat: 2g
- Sodium: 200mg

Serves: 4 Cooking Time: 20 minutes

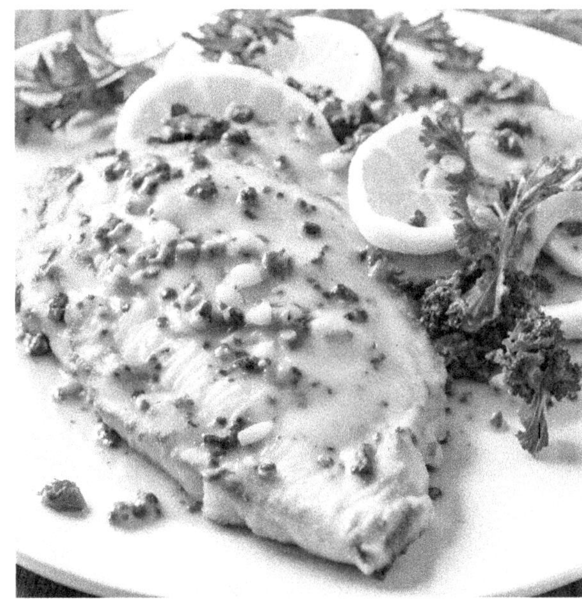

16. Herb Roasted Chicken Thighs

Ingredients:

- 8 bone-in, skin-on chicken thighs
- 1/4 cup olive oil
- 2 tablespoons fresh rosemary, chopped
- 2 tablespoons fresh thyme, chopped
- 2 garlic cloves, minced
- 1 lemon, zested and juiced
- 1/2 teaspoon paprika

Instructions:

1. Preheat the oven to 400°F (200°C). Line a baking sheet with parchment paper.
2. In a small bowl, mix the olive oil, rosemary, thyme, minced garlic, lemon zest, lemon juice, and paprika.
3. Rub the herb mixture all over the chicken thighs, making sure to get some under the skin.
4. Place the chicken thighs on the prepared baking sheet.
5. Roast in the preheated oven for 35-40 minutes, until the chicken is cooked through and the skin is crispy.
6. Serve immediately.

Nutrition Info (per serving):

- Calories: 350
- Protein: 30g
- Carbohydrates: 3g
- Dietary Fiber: 1g
- Sugars: 0g
- Fat: 24g
- Saturated Fat: 6g
- Sodium: 120mg

Serves: 4 Cooking Time: 40 minutes

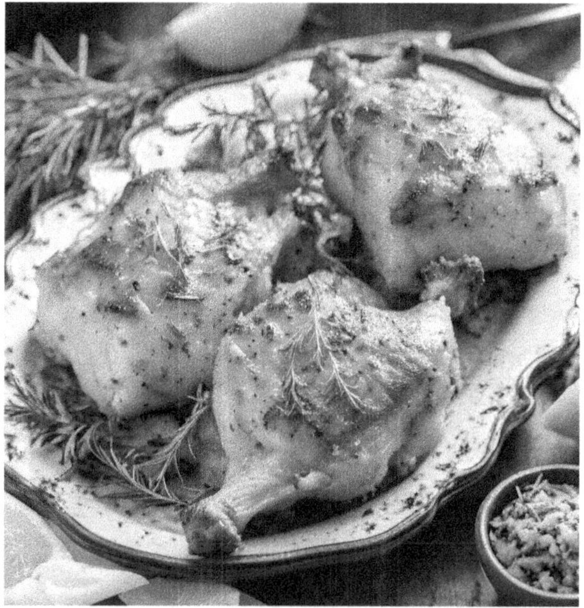

17. Chicken and Broccoli Stir-Fry

Ingredients:

- 1 pound boneless, skinless chicken breasts, sliced into thin strips
- 3 cups broccoli florets
- 2 tablespoons olive oil
- 1 medium onion, sliced
- 3 garlic cloves, minced
- 1 tablespoon fresh ginger, grated
- 1/4 cup low-sodium soy sauce
- 2 tablespoons rice vinegar
- 1 tablespoon honey
- 1 teaspoon sesame oil
- 1 tablespoon sesame seeds (optional)
- 1/4 cup fresh cilantro, chopped (optional)

Instructions:

1. In a small bowl, whisk together the soy sauce, rice vinegar, honey, and sesame oil. Set aside.
2. Heat 1 tablespoon of olive oil in a large skillet or wok over medium-high heat.
3. Add the chicken strips and cook until browned and cooked through, about 5-7 minutes. Remove the chicken from the skillet and set aside.
4. In the same skillet, add the remaining olive oil. Add the sliced onion and cook until softened, about 3 minutes.
5. Add the minced garlic and grated ginger, and cook for another 1-2 minutes.
6. Add the broccoli florets and stir-fry for about 5 minutes until they are tender but still crisp.
7. Return the chicken to the skillet and pour the soy sauce mixture over everything. Stir to combine and cook for another 2-3 minutes until heated through.
8. Serve immediately, garnished with sesame seeds and fresh cilantro if desired.

Nutrition Info (per serving):

- Calories: 280
- Protein: 28g
- Carbohydrates: 15g
- Dietary Fiber: 4g
- Sugars: 7g
- Fat: 12g
- Saturated Fat: 2g
- Sodium: 450mg

Serves: 4 Cooking Time: 20 minutes

18. Garlic Lemon Turkey Cutlets

Ingredients:

- 4 turkey cutlets (about 4 ounces each)
- 2 tablespoons olive oil
- 3 garlic cloves, minced
- 1 lemon, zested and juiced
- 1 teaspoon dried oregano
- 1/4 cup low-sodium chicken broth
- 1 tablespoon fresh parsley, chopped

Instructions:

1. Heat the olive oil in a large skillet over medium-high heat.
2. Add the turkey cutlets and cook for 3-4 minutes on each side, until golden brown and cooked through. Remove the cutlets from the skillet and set aside.
3. In the same skillet, add the minced garlic and cook for about 1 minute until fragrant.
4. Add the lemon juice, lemon zest, dried oregano, and chicken broth. Bring to a simmer and cook for 2-3 minutes until the sauce thickens slightly.
5. Return the turkey cutlets to the skillet and coat them with the sauce.
6. Garnish with fresh parsley before serving.

Nutrition Info (per serving):

- Calories: 220
- Protein: 26g
- Carbohydrates: 4g
- Dietary Fiber: 1g
- Sugars: 1g
- Fat: 10g
- Saturated Fat: 1.5g
- Sodium: 150mg

Serves: 4 Cooking Time: 15 minutes

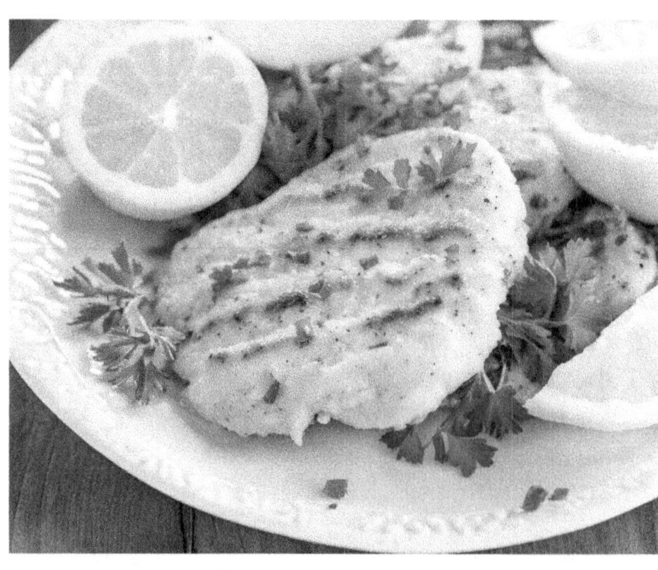

19. Chicken Curry with Coconut Milk

Ingredients:

- 1 pound boneless, skinless chicken thighs, cut into bite-sized pieces
- 2 tablespoons olive oil
- 1 large onion, chopped
- 3 garlic cloves, minced
- 1 tablespoon fresh ginger, grated
- 2 tablespoons curry powder
- 1 can (14 ounces) coconut milk (unsweetened)
- 1 cup low-sodium chicken broth
- 1 cup diced tomatoes (canned or fresh)
- 1 cup carrots, sliced
- 1 cup green beans, trimmed and cut into 1-inch pieces
- 1/4 cup fresh cilantro, chopped

Instructions:

1. Heat the olive oil in a large pot over medium heat.
2. Add the chopped onion and cook until softened, about 5 minutes.
3. Add the minced garlic and grated ginger, and cook for another 1-2 minutes until fragrant.
4. Stir in the curry powder and cook for 1 minute.
5. Add the chicken pieces and cook until browned, about 5-7 minutes.
6. Pour in the coconut milk and chicken broth, and stir to combine.
7. Add the diced tomatoes, carrots, and green beans. Bring to a simmer and cook for 20-25 minutes, until the vegetables are tender and the chicken is cooked through.
8. Garnish with fresh cilantro before serving.

Nutrition Info (per serving):

- Calories: 350
- Protein: 28g
- Carbohydrates: 15g
- Dietary Fiber: 4g
- Sugars: 6g
- Fat: 20g
- Saturated Fat: 10g
- Sodium: 300mg

Serves: 4 Cooking Time: 35 minutes

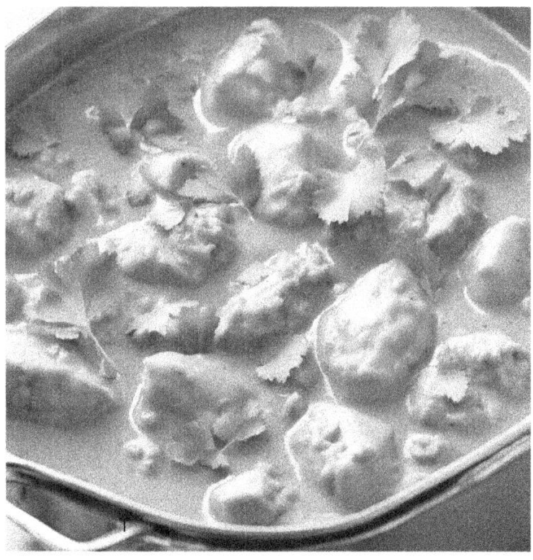

20. Smoked Turkey Breast

Ingredients:

- 1 whole turkey breast (about 4-5 pounds)
- 1/4 cup olive oil
- 2 tablespoons apple cider vinegar
- 2 garlic cloves, minced
- 1 tablespoon smoked paprika
- 1 teaspoon dried thyme
- 1 teaspoon dried rosemary
- 1/2 teaspoon cumin

Instructions:

1. In a small bowl, mix the olive oil, apple cider vinegar, minced garlic, smoked paprika, thyme, rosemary, and cumin.
2. Rub the mixture all over the turkey breast, making sure to get some under the skin.
3. Preheat the smoker to 225°F (110°C).
4. Place the turkey breast in the smoker and smoke for about 3-4 hours, until the internal temperature reaches 165°F (74°C).
5. Remove the turkey breast from the smoker and let it rest for 10-15 minutes before slicing.
6. Serve immediately.

Nutrition Info (per serving):

- Calories: 320
- Protein: 42g
- Carbohydrates: 2g
- Dietary Fiber: 1g
- Sugars: 0g
- Fat: 16g
- Saturated Fat: 3g
- Sodium: 180mg

Serves: 8 Cooking Time: 4 hours

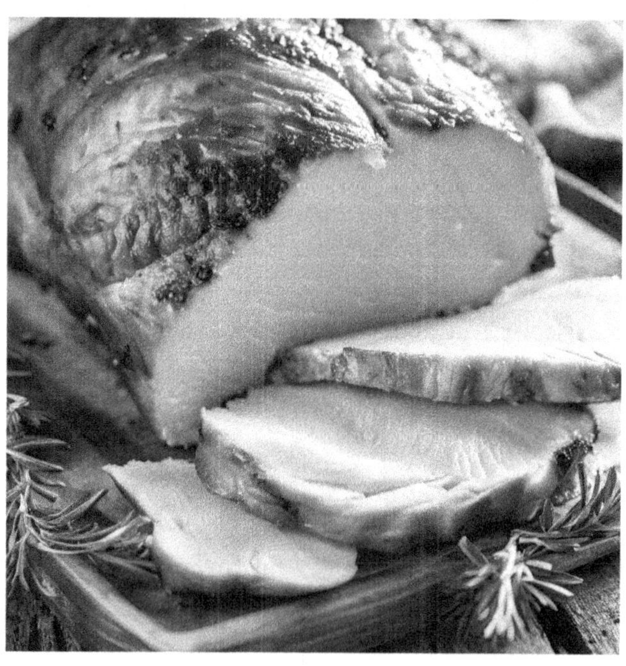

21. Turkey Meatloaf with Spinach

Ingredients:

- 1 pound ground turkey
- 1 cup fresh spinach, finely chopped
- 1/2 cup whole wheat breadcrumbs
- 1/4 cup grated Parmesan cheese
- 1 egg, beaten
- 1 small onion, finely chopped
- 2 garlic cloves, minced
- 1 tablespoon Worcestershire sauce
- 1 tablespoon olive oil
- 1/2 teaspoon dried thyme
- 1/2 teaspoon dried oregano

Instructions:

1. Preheat the oven to 375°F (190°C). Grease a loaf pan with olive oil.
2. In a large bowl, mix the ground turkey, chopped spinach, breadcrumbs, Parmesan cheese, beaten egg, chopped onion, minced garlic, Worcestershire sauce, olive oil, thyme, and oregano until well combined.
3. Transfer the mixture to the prepared loaf pan and press down gently to shape it.
4. Bake in the preheated oven for 45-50 minutes, until the meatloaf is cooked through and reaches an internal temperature of 165°F (74°C).
5. Let the meatloaf rest for 10 minutes before slicing and serving.

Nutrition Info (per serving):

- Calories: 220
- Protein: 22g
- Carbohydrates: 10g
- Dietary Fiber: 2g
- Sugars: 2g
- Fat: 10g
- Saturated Fat: 2g
- Sodium: 320mg

Serves: 4 Cooking Time: 50 minutes

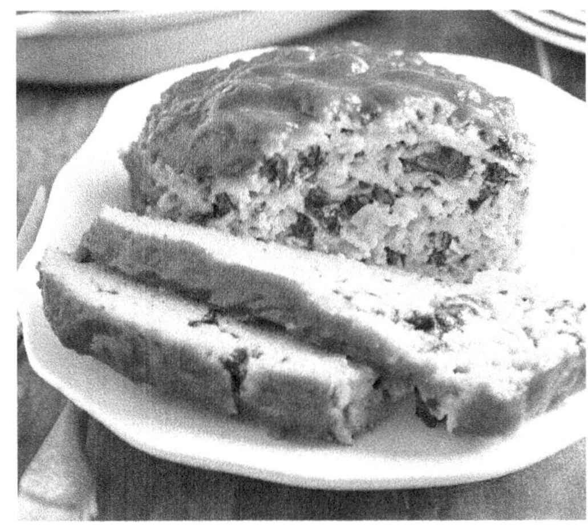

22. Balsamic Glazed Turkey Drumsticks

Ingredients:

- 4 turkey drumsticks
- 1/4 cup balsamic vinegar
- 2 tablespoons honey
- 2 tablespoons olive oil
- 3 garlic cloves, minced
- 1 teaspoon dried rosemary
- 1 teaspoon dried thyme

Instructions:

1. Preheat the oven to 375°F (190°C). Line a baking sheet with parchment paper.
2. In a small bowl, mix the balsamic vinegar, honey, olive oil, minced garlic, rosemary, and thyme.
3. Place the turkey drumsticks on the prepared baking sheet and brush them with the balsamic mixture.
4. Roast in the preheated oven for 50-60 minutes, basting occasionally with the remaining glaze, until the drumsticks are cooked through and reach an internal temperature of 165°F (74°C).
5. Let the drumsticks rest for 10 minutes before serving.

Nutrition Info (per serving):

- Calories: 350
- Protein: 35g
- Carbohydrates: 12g
- Dietary Fiber: 1g
- Sugars: 10g
- Fat: 18g
- Saturated Fat: 4g
- Sodium: 240mg

Serves: 4 Cooking Time: 1 hour

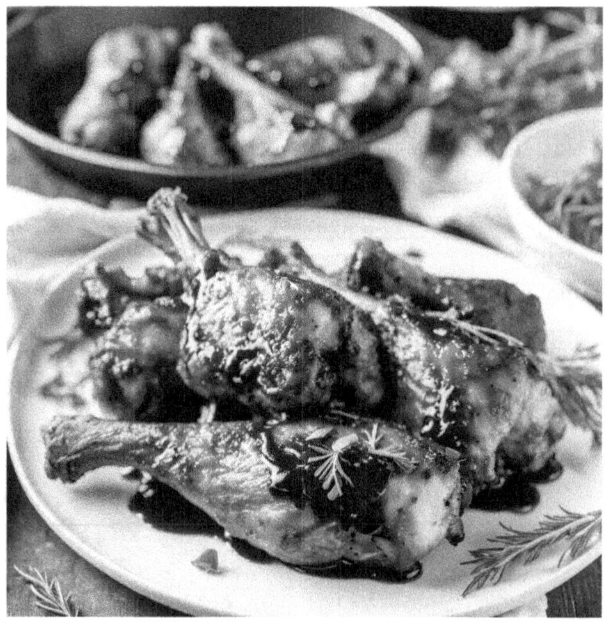

23. Turkey Bolognese over Zucchini Noodles

Ingredients:

- 1 pound ground turkey
- 3 medium zucchinis, spiralized into noodles
- 2 tablespoons olive oil
- 1 large onion, chopped
- 3 garlic cloves, minced
- 1 carrot, finely chopped
- 1 celery stalk, finely chopped
- 1 can (14.5 ounces) diced tomatoes, with juice
- 1/4 cup tomato paste
- 1/2 cup low-sodium chicken broth
- 1 teaspoon dried basil
- 1 teaspoon dried oregano
- 1/4 cup fresh parsley, chopped

Instructions:

1. Heat 1 tablespoon of olive oil in a large skillet over medium-high heat.
2. Add the ground turkey and cook until browned, about 7-8 minutes. Remove the turkey from the skillet and set aside.
3. In the same skillet, add the remaining olive oil. Add the chopped onion, garlic, carrot, and celery, and cook until softened, about 5 minutes.
4. Stir in the diced tomatoes, tomato paste, chicken broth, basil, and oregano. Return the ground turkey to the skillet and bring to a simmer.
5. Cook for 20-25 minutes, until the sauce thickens and the flavors meld together.
6. While the sauce is cooking, heat a separate skillet over medium heat. Add the spiralized zucchini noodles and cook for 3-4 minutes, until just tender.
7. Serve the turkey Bolognese sauce over the zucchini noodles, garnished with fresh parsley.

Nutrition Info (per serving):

- Calories: 280
- Protein: 28g
- Carbohydrates: 15g
- Dietary Fiber: 5g
- Sugars: 8g
- Fat: 12g
- Saturated Fat: 2g
- Sodium: 350mg

Serves: 4 Cooking Time: 35 minutes

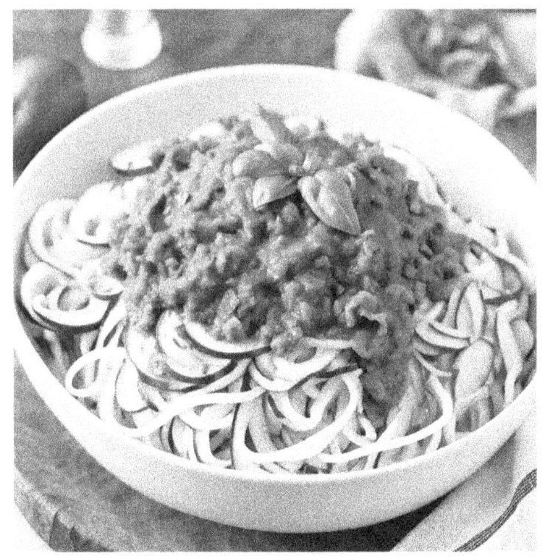

24. Chicken Pot Pie with Phyllo Crust

Ingredients:

- 1 pound boneless, skinless chicken breasts, cubed
- 2 tablespoons olive oil
- 1 large onion, chopped
- 2 garlic cloves, minced
- 2 cups low-sodium chicken broth
- 1 cup carrots, diced
- 1 cup peas
- 1 cup celery, diced
- 1/2 cup unsweetened almond milk
- 2 tablespoons whole wheat flour
- 1 teaspoon dried thyme
- 8 sheets phyllo dough
- 1 tablespoon olive oil (for brushing)

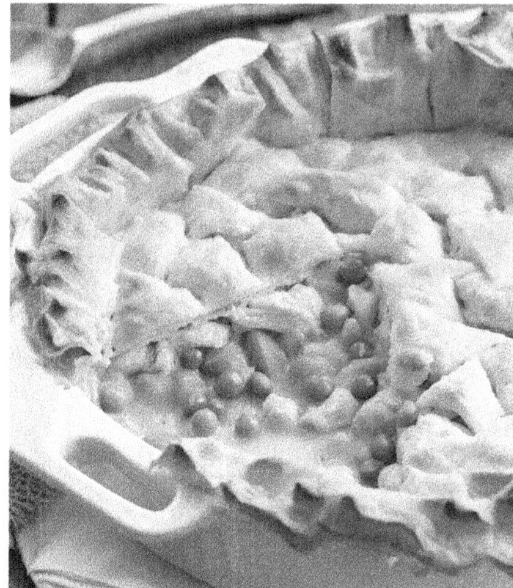

Instructions:

1. Preheat the oven to 375°F (190°C).
2. Heat the olive oil in a large skillet over medium-high heat. Add the cubed chicken and cook until browned and cooked through, about 7-8 minutes. Remove the chicken from the skillet and set aside.
3. In the same skillet, add the chopped onion and minced garlic, and cook until softened, about 5 minutes.
4. Stir in the whole wheat flour and cook for 1 minute.
5. Gradually add the chicken broth and almond milk, stirring constantly, until the mixture thickens, about 5 minutes.
6. Add the carrots, peas, celery, cooked chicken, and dried thyme. Cook for another 5 minutes until the vegetables are tender.
7. Transfer the mixture to a baking dish.
8. Layer the phyllo sheets over the filling, brushing each sheet with olive oil before adding the next.
9. Bake in the preheated oven for 20-25 minutes, until the phyllo crust is golden and crisp.
10. Serve immediately.

Nutrition Info (per serving):

- Calories: 320 Protein: 26g Carbohydrates: 25g Dietary Fiber: 5g
- Sugars: 6g Fat: 12g Saturated Fat: 2g
- Sodium: 280mg

Serves: 4 Cooking Time: 35 minutes

25. Roasted Chicken with Squash and Cranberries

Ingredients:

- 4 bone-in, skin-on chicken thighs
- 2 tablespoons olive oil
- 2 cups butternut squash, cubed
- 1 cup fresh cranberries
- 1 tablespoon honey
- 1 teaspoon dried rosemary
- 1 teaspoon dried thyme

Instructions:

1. Preheat the oven to 400°F (200°C). Line a baking sheet with parchment paper.
2. In a small bowl, mix the olive oil, honey, rosemary, and thyme.
3. Place the chicken thighs on the prepared baking sheet and brush them with the olive oil mixture.
4. Arrange the cubed butternut squash and cranberries around the chicken thighs.
5. Roast in the preheated oven for 35-40 minutes, until the chicken is cooked through and the skin is crispy, and the squash is tender.
6. Serve immediately.

Nutrition Info (per serving):

- Calories: 380
- Protein: 28g
- Carbohydrates: 20g
- Dietary Fiber: 5g
- Sugars: 8g
- Fat: 22g
- Saturated Fat: 5g
- Sodium: 180mg

Serves: 4 Cooking Time: 40 minutes

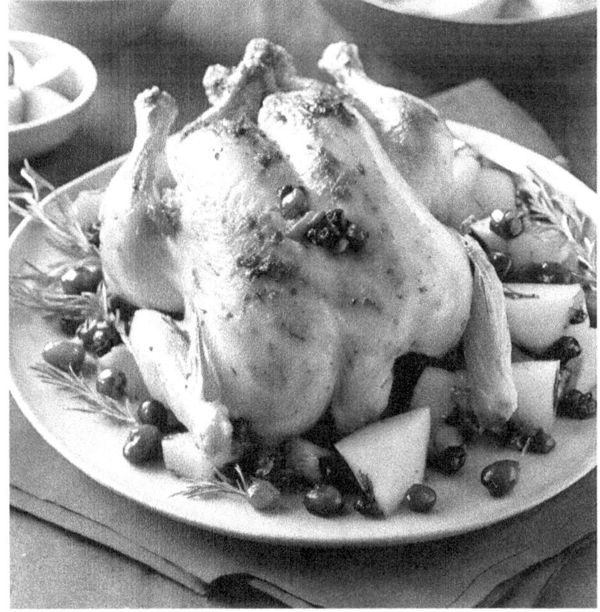

Vegetables

1. Roasted Brussels Sprouts with Balsamic Glaze
Ingredients:
- 1 pound Brussels sprouts, trimmed and halved
- 2 tablespoons olive oil
- 2 tablespoons balsamic vinegar
- 1 tablespoon honey
- 1/4 cup dried cranberries
- 1/4 cup chopped walnuts (optional)

Instructions:
1. Preheat the oven to 400°F (200°C). Line a baking sheet with parchment paper.
2. In a large bowl, toss the Brussels sprouts with olive oil until evenly coated.
3. Spread the Brussels sprouts on the prepared baking sheet in a single layer.
4. Roast in the preheated oven for 20-25 minutes, until the Brussels sprouts are golden and crispy on the edges.
5. Meanwhile, in a small saucepan, combine the balsamic vinegar and honey. Simmer over medium heat for 5-7 minutes until the mixture has thickened to a glaze.
6. Drizzle the balsamic glaze over the roasted Brussels sprouts and sprinkle with dried cranberries and chopped walnuts (if using).
7. Serve immediately.

Nutrition Info (per serving):
- Calories: 140
- Protein: 3g
- Carbohydrates: 18g
- Dietary Fiber: 4g
- Sugars: 10g
- Fat: 7g
- Saturated Fat: 1g
- Sodium: 40mg

Serves: 4 Cooking Time: 30 minutes

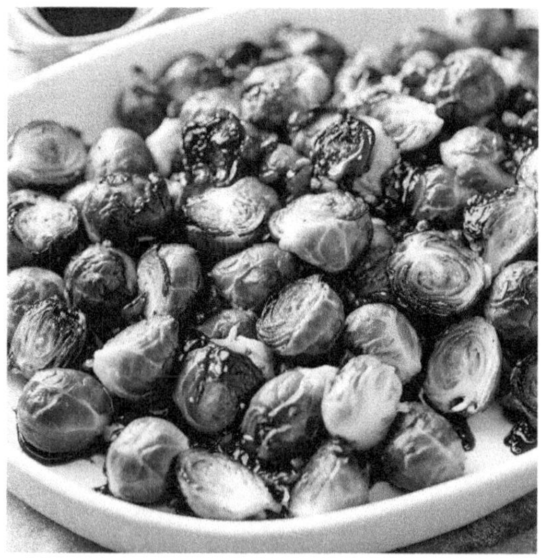

2. Carrot Ginger Soup

Ingredients:

- 1 tablespoon olive oil
- 1 large onion, chopped
- 2 garlic cloves, minced
- 1 tablespoon fresh ginger, grated
- 1 pound carrots, peeled and chopped
- 4 cups low-sodium vegetable broth
- 1 cup unsweetened coconut milk
- 1 tablespoon fresh lemon juice
- 1/4 cup fresh cilantro, chopped (for garnish)

Instructions:

1. Heat the olive oil in a large pot over medium heat.
2. Add the chopped onion and cook until softened, about 5 minutes.
3. Add the minced garlic and grated ginger, and cook for another 1-2 minutes until fragrant.
4. Add the chopped carrots and vegetable broth. Bring to a boil, then reduce the heat and simmer for 20-25 minutes until the carrots are tender.
5. Using an immersion blender, blend the soup until smooth. Alternatively, transfer the soup to a blender in batches and blend until smooth.
6. Stir in the coconut milk and fresh lemon juice.
7. Serve the soup hot, garnished with fresh cilantro.

Nutrition Info (per serving):

- Calories: 160
- Protein: 2g
- Carbohydrates: 18g
- Dietary Fiber: 4g
- Sugars: 9g
- Fat: 9g
- Saturated Fat: 7g
- Sodium: 300mg

Serves: 4 Cooking Time: 30 minutes

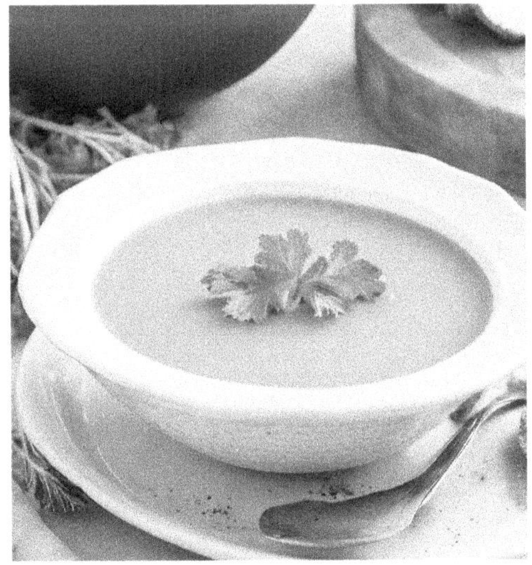

3. Spiced Sweet Potato Wedges

Ingredients:

- 2 large sweet potatoes, cut into wedges
- 2 tablespoons olive oil
- 1 teaspoon ground cumin
- 1 teaspoon paprika
- 1/2 teaspoon ground cinnamon
- 1 tablespoon honey
- 1 tablespoon fresh lime juice

Instructions:

1. Preheat the oven to 400°F (200°C). Line a baking sheet with parchment paper.
2. In a large bowl, toss the sweet potato wedges with olive oil, ground cumin, paprika, and ground cinnamon until evenly coated.
3. Spread the sweet potato wedges on the prepared baking sheet in a single layer.
4. Roast in the preheated oven for 25-30 minutes, turning halfway through, until the wedges are tender and golden brown.
5. Drizzle the honey and fresh lime juice over the roasted sweet potato wedges before serving.
6. Serve immediately.

Nutrition Info (per serving):

- Calories: 180
- Protein: 2g
- Carbohydrates: 28g
- Dietary Fiber: 5g
- Sugars: 10g
- Fat: 7g
- Saturated Fat: 1g
- Sodium: 50mg

Serves: 4 Cooking Time: 30 minutes

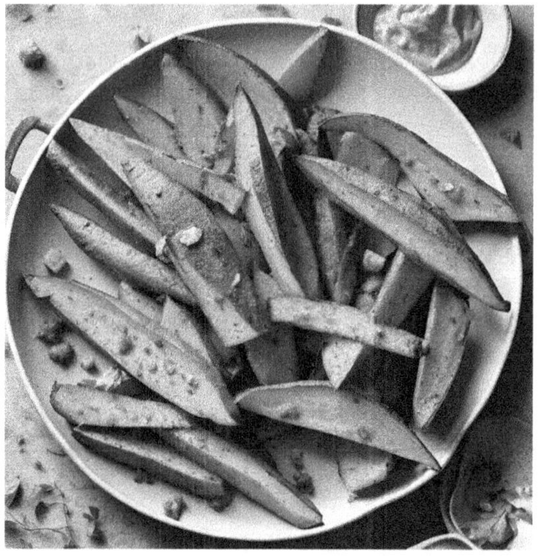

4. Beet and Goat Cheese Salad

Ingredients:

- 4 medium beets, roasted, peeled, and sliced
- 4 cups mixed greens (arugula, spinach, and/or kale)
- 1/4 cup goat cheese, crumbled
- 1/4 cup walnuts, toasted and chopped
- 2 tablespoons balsamic vinegar
- 1 tablespoon olive oil
- 1 teaspoon honey

Instructions:

1. Preheat the oven to 400°F (200°C). Wrap each beet in aluminum foil and place them on a baking sheet. Roast for 45-60 minutes, until tender. Allow to cool, then peel and slice the beets.
2. In a small bowl, whisk together the balsamic vinegar, olive oil, and honey to make the dressing.
3. In a large bowl, combine the mixed greens, sliced beets, crumbled goat cheese, and toasted walnuts.
4. Drizzle the dressing over the salad and toss gently to combine.
5. Serve immediately.

Nutrition Info (per serving):

- Calories: 180
- Protein: 5g
- Carbohydrates: 18g
- Dietary Fiber: 4g
- Sugars: 12g
- Fat: 10g
- Saturated Fat: 2g
- Sodium: 130mg

Serves: 4 Cooking Time: 60 minutes

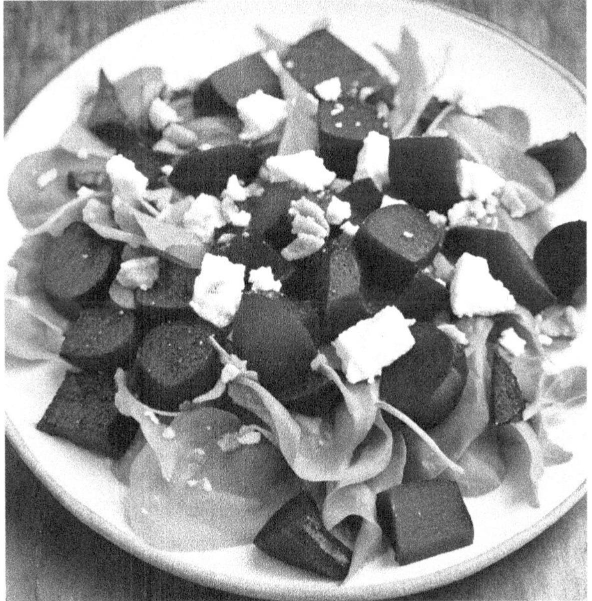

5. Cauliflower Steak with Herb Sauce

Ingredients:

- 1 large head of cauliflower
- 3 tablespoons olive oil, divided
- 2 tablespoons fresh parsley, chopped
- 1 tablespoon fresh thyme, chopped
- 1 tablespoon fresh rosemary, chopped
- 1 garlic clove, minced
- 1 tablespoon lemon juice
- 1 teaspoon Dijon mustard

Instructions:

1. Preheat the oven to 400°F (200°C). Line a baking sheet with parchment paper.
2. Remove the outer leaves of the cauliflower and trim the stem. Slice the cauliflower into 1-inch thick steaks.
3. Brush both sides of the cauliflower steaks with 2 tablespoons of olive oil.
4. Arrange the cauliflower steaks on the prepared baking sheet and roast in the preheated oven for 25-30 minutes, until golden brown and tender, flipping halfway through.
5. While the cauliflower is roasting, prepare the herb sauce. In a small bowl, combine the remaining olive oil, chopped parsley, thyme, rosemary, minced garlic, lemon juice, and Dijon mustard. Mix well.
6. Drizzle the herb sauce over the roasted cauliflower steaks before serving.
7. Serve immediately.

Nutrition Info (per serving):

- Calories: 140
- Protein: 3g
- Carbohydrates: 12g
- Dietary Fiber: 4g
- Sugars: 4g
- Fat: 10g
- Saturated Fat: 1.5g
- Sodium: 100mg

Serves: 4 Cooking Time: 30 minutes

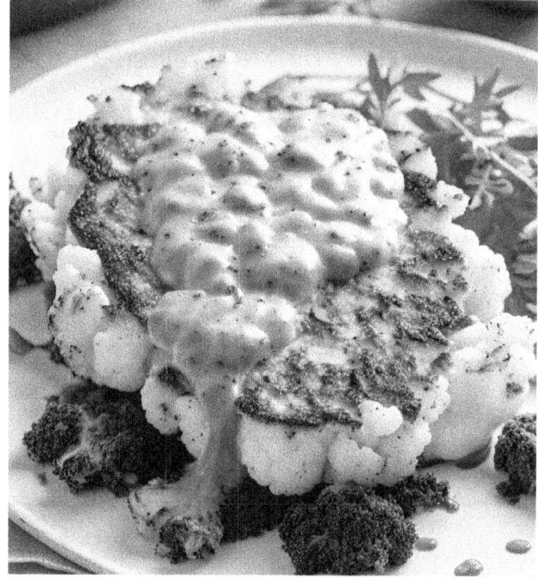

6. Butternut Squash Risotto

Ingredients:

- 1 cup Arborio rice
- 2 tablespoons olive oil
- 1 small onion, finely chopped
- 2 garlic cloves, minced
- 3 cups low-sodium vegetable broth, warmed
- 2 cups butternut squash, peeled and diced
- 1/2 cup dry white wine (optional)
- 1/4 cup Parmesan cheese, grated
- 2 tablespoons fresh parsley, chopped

Instructions:

1. Heat the olive oil in a large saucepan over medium heat.
2. Add the finely chopped onion and cook until softened, about 5 minutes.
3. Add the minced garlic and cook for another 1-2 minutes.
4. Stir in the Arborio rice and cook for 1-2 minutes until the rice is lightly toasted.
5. If using, pour in the white wine and cook until it has mostly evaporated.
6. Gradually add the warmed vegetable broth, one ladleful at a time, stirring constantly and allowing each addition to be absorbed before adding more.
7. After about 10 minutes, add the diced butternut squash to the risotto.
8. Continue to cook, adding broth as needed, until the rice is creamy and the butternut squash is tender, about 20-25 minutes total.
9. Stir in the grated Parmesan cheese and chopped parsley.
10. Serve immediately.

Nutrition Info (per serving):

- Calories: 270
- Protein: 6g
- Carbohydrates: 44g
- Dietary Fiber: 4g
- Sugars: 4g
- Fat: 8g
- Saturated Fat: 2g
- Sodium: 220mg

Serves: 4 Cooking Time: 30 minutes

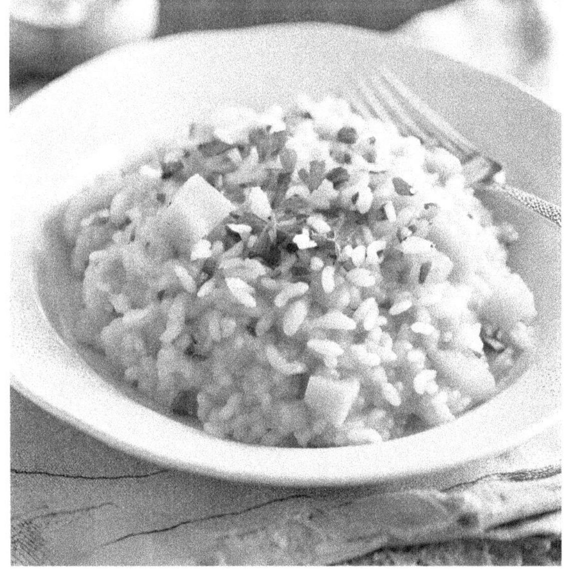

7. **Sauteed Green Beans with Garlic**

Ingredients:

- 1 pound fresh green beans, trimmed
- 2 tablespoons olive oil
- 4 garlic cloves, thinly sliced
- 1 tablespoon lemon juice
- 1/4 cup slivered almonds, toasted (optional)

Instructions:

1. Bring a large pot of water to a boil. Add the green beans and blanch for 3-4 minutes until tender-crisp. Drain and set aside.
2. Heat the olive oil in a large skillet over medium heat.
3. Add the sliced garlic and cook for 1-2 minutes until fragrant and lightly golden.
4. Add the blanched green beans to the skillet and sauté for 4-5 minutes until heated through and coated with the garlic oil.
5. Stir in the lemon juice and cook for another 1 minute.
6. If using, sprinkle the toasted slivered almonds over the green beans before serving.
7. Serve immediately.

Nutrition Info (per serving):

- Calories: 110
- Protein: 3g
- Carbohydrates: 10g
- Dietary Fiber: 4g
- Sugars: 4g
- Fat: 7g
- Saturated Fat: 1g
- Sodium: 10mg

Serves: 4 Cooking Time: 15 minutes

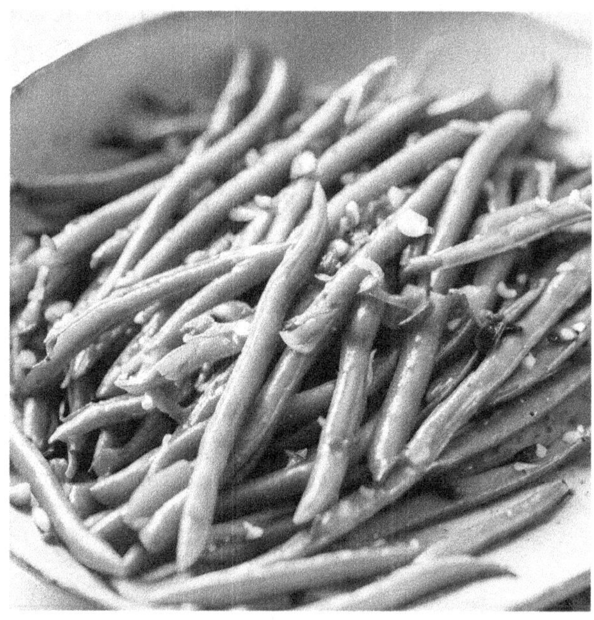

8. Eggplant Parmesan Stacks

Ingredients:

- 2 large eggplants, sliced into 1/2-inch rounds
- 2 tablespoons olive oil
- 1 cup marinara sauce (low sodium)
- 1 cup shredded mozzarella cheese
- 1/4 cup grated Parmesan cheese
- 1/4 cup fresh basil leaves, chopped

Instructions:

1. Preheat the oven to 375°F (190°C). Line a baking sheet with parchment paper.
2. Brush both sides of the eggplant slices with olive oil and arrange them on the prepared baking sheet.
3. Bake in the preheated oven for 20 minutes, flipping halfway through, until the eggplant is tender and golden brown.
4. Spread a thin layer of marinara sauce on the bottom of a baking dish.
5. Place a layer of eggplant slices on top of the sauce, followed by a layer of marinara sauce, shredded mozzarella, and a sprinkle of grated Parmesan.
6. Repeat the layers until all the eggplant slices are used, ending with a layer of cheese on top.
7. Bake in the preheated oven for 20-25 minutes, until the cheese is melted and bubbly.
8. Garnish with chopped fresh basil before serving.
9. Serve immediately.

Nutrition Info (per serving):

- Calories: 220
- Protein: 10g
- Carbohydrates: 20g
- Dietary Fiber: 7g
- Sugars: 9g
- Fat: 12g
- Saturated Fat: 4g
- Sodium: 260mg

Serves: 4 Cooking Time: 45 minutes

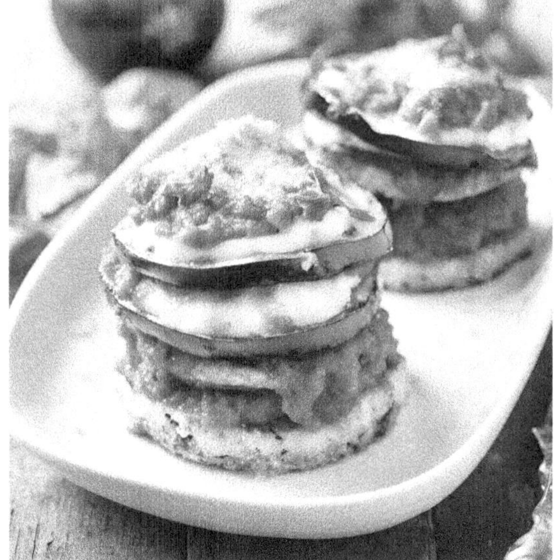

9. Spaghetti Squash with Tomato Sauce

Ingredients:

- 1 medium spaghetti squash
- 2 tablespoons olive oil
- 1 onion, chopped
- 3 garlic cloves, minced
- 1 can (14.5 ounces) diced tomatoes, with juice
- 1 teaspoon dried oregano
- 1 teaspoon dried basil
- 1/4 teaspoon red pepper flakes (optional)
- 1/4 cup fresh parsley, chopped
- 1/4 cup grated Parmesan cheese (optional)

Instructions:

1. Preheat the oven to 375°F (190°C). Line a baking sheet with parchment paper.
2. Cut the spaghetti squash in half lengthwise and remove the seeds. Brush the inside with 1 tablespoon of olive oil.
3. Place the squash halves, cut side down, on the prepared baking sheet and bake for 35-40 minutes until tender.
4. While the squash is baking, heat the remaining olive oil in a large skillet over medium heat. Add the chopped onion and cook until softened, about 5 minutes.
5. Add the minced garlic and cook for another 1-2 minutes.
6. Stir in the diced tomatoes, oregano, basil, and red pepper flakes (if using). Simmer for 15-20 minutes until the sauce thickens.
7. When the squash is done, use a fork to scrape out the flesh into strands.
8. Serve the spaghetti squash topped with the tomato sauce, fresh parsley, and grated Parmesan cheese (if using).

Nutrition Info (per serving):

- Calories: 150
- Protein: 3g
- Carbohydrates: 18g
- Dietary Fiber: 4g
- Sugars: 8g
- Fat: 8g
- Saturated Fat: 1g
- Sodium: 100mg

Serves: 4 Cooking Time: 45 minutes

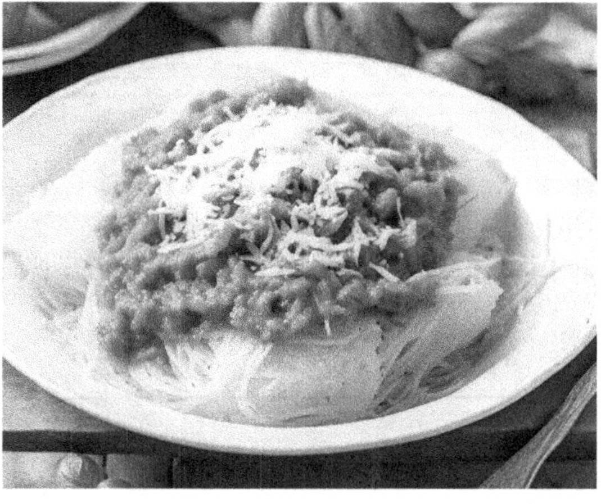

10. Creamed Spinach

Ingredients:

- 2 tablespoons olive oil
- 1 small onion, finely chopped
- 2 garlic cloves, minced
- 1 pound fresh spinach, washed and chopped
- 1 cup unsweetened almond milk
- 1 tablespoon whole wheat flour
- 1/4 teaspoon ground nutmeg
- 1/4 cup grated Parmesan cheese (optional)

Instructions:

1. Heat the olive oil in a large skillet over medium heat.
2. Add the finely chopped onion and cook until softened, about 5 minutes.
3. Add the minced garlic and cook for another 1-2 minutes.
4. Add the chopped spinach and cook until wilted, about 3-4 minutes.
5. In a small bowl, whisk together the almond milk and whole wheat flour until smooth. Pour the mixture into the skillet with the spinach.
6. Stir in the ground nutmeg and cook for another 2-3 minutes until the mixture thickens.
7. If using, stir in the grated Parmesan cheese until melted.
8. Serve immediately.

Nutrition Info (per serving):

- Calories: 110
- Protein: 4g
- Carbohydrates: 8g
- Dietary Fiber: 3g
- Sugars: 2g
- Fat: 8g
- Saturated Fat: 1.5g
- Sodium: 80mg

Serves: 4 Cooking Time: 20 minutes

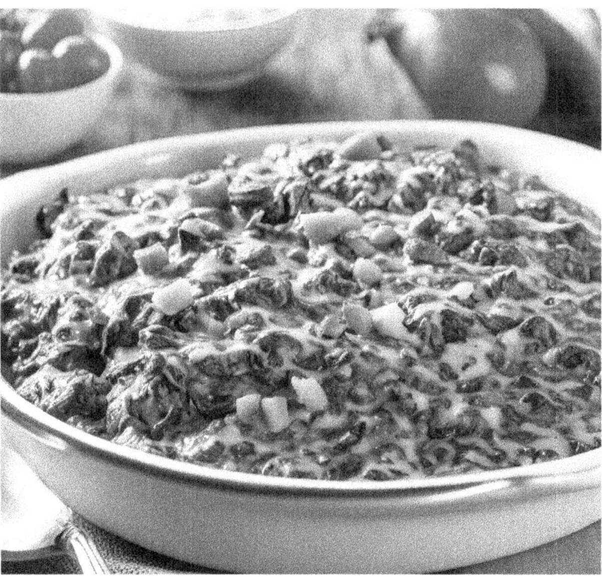

11. Broccoli and Cashew Stir-Fry

Ingredients:

- 2 tablespoons olive oil
- 1 pound broccoli florets
- 1 red bell pepper, sliced
- 3 garlic cloves, minced
- 1 tablespoon fresh ginger, grated
- 1/4 cup low-sodium soy sauce
- 2 tablespoons rice vinegar
- 1 tablespoon honey
- 1/4 cup cashews, toasted
- 1 tablespoon sesame seeds (optional)

Instructions:

1. Heat the olive oil in a large skillet or wok over medium-high heat.
2. Add the broccoli florets and red bell pepper slices, and stir-fry for 5-7 minutes until tender-crisp.
3. Add the minced garlic and grated ginger, and cook for another 1-2 minutes until fragrant.
4. In a small bowl, whisk together the soy sauce, rice vinegar, and honey. Pour the sauce over the vegetables in the skillet.
5. Stir in the toasted cashews and cook for another 2-3 minutes until everything is well coated and heated through.
6. If using, sprinkle the stir-fry with sesame seeds before serving.
7. Serve immediately.

Nutrition Info (per serving):

- Calories: 180
- Protein: 5g
- Carbohydrates: 15g
- Dietary Fiber: 4g
- Sugars: 6g
- Fat: 12g
- Saturated Fat: 2g
- Sodium: 360mg

Serves: 4 Cooking Time: 15 minutes

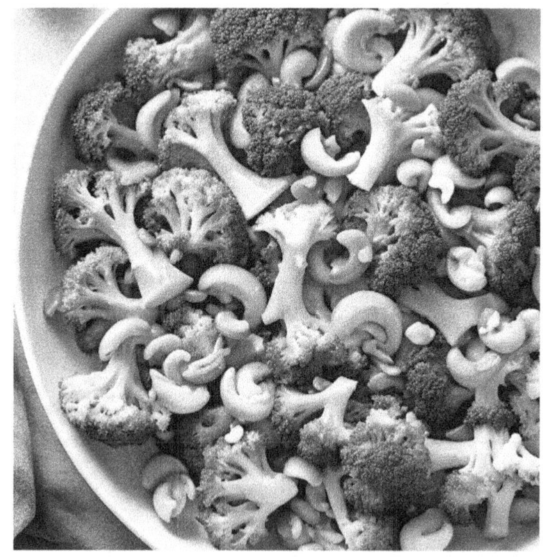

12. Kale Salad with Avocado and Pomegranate

Ingredients:

- 6 cups kale, washed and chopped
- 1 avocado, diced
- 1/2 cup pomegranate seeds
- 1/4 cup walnuts, toasted and chopped
- 2 tablespoons olive oil
- 1 tablespoon lemon juice
- 1 teaspoon Dijon mustard

Instructions:

1. In a large bowl, massage the chopped kale with 1 tablespoon of olive oil until it becomes tender, about 2-3 minutes.
2. In a small bowl, whisk together the remaining olive oil, lemon juice, and Dijon mustard to make the dressing.
3. Add the diced avocado, pomegranate seeds, and toasted walnuts to the kale.
4. Pour the dressing over the salad and toss to combine.
5. Serve immediately.

Nutrition Info (per serving):

- Calories: 220
- Protein: 4g
- Carbohydrates: 14g
- Dietary Fiber: 6g
- Sugars: 5g
- Fat: 18g
- Saturated Fat: 2.5g
- Sodium: 60mg

Serves: 4 Cooking Time: 10 minutes

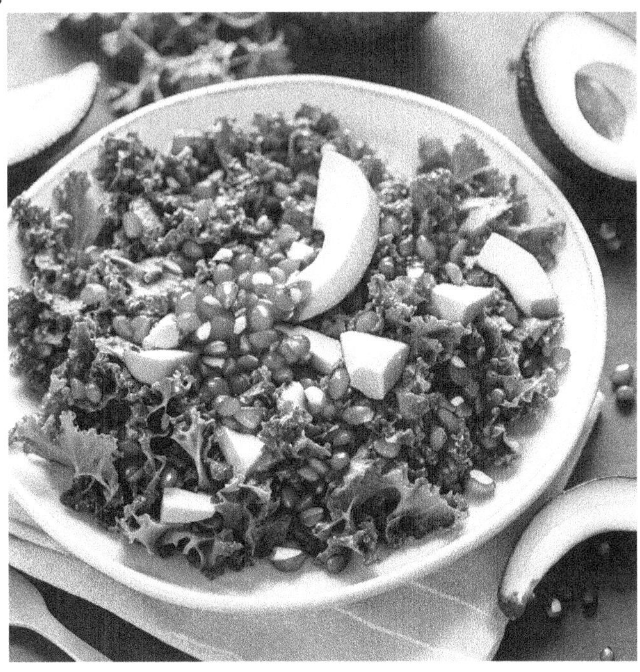

13. Mushroom and Barley Pilaf

Ingredients:

- 1 cup pearl barley, rinsed
- 2 tablespoons olive oil
- 1 onion, finely chopped
- 2 garlic cloves, minced
- 2 cups mushrooms, sliced
- 4 cups low-sodium vegetable broth
- 1 teaspoon dried thyme
- 1/4 cup fresh parsley, chopped

Instructions:

1. Heat the olive oil in a large pot over medium heat.
2. Add the chopped onion and cook until softened, about 5 minutes.
3. Add the minced garlic and sliced mushrooms, and cook for another 5-7 minutes until the mushrooms are tender.
4. Stir in the rinsed barley and cook for 2 minutes, coating the barley with the oil and vegetables.
5. Add the vegetable broth and dried thyme, and bring to a boil.
6. Reduce the heat to low, cover, and simmer for 40-45 minutes, until the barley is tender and the liquid is absorbed.
7. Stir in the chopped parsley before serving.
8. Serve immediately.

Nutrition Info (per serving):

- Calories: 220
- Protein: 6g
- Carbohydrates: 42g
- Dietary Fiber: 8g
- Sugars: 4g
- Fat: 6g
- Saturated Fat: 1g
- Sodium: 150mg

Serves: 4 Cooking Time: 50 minutes

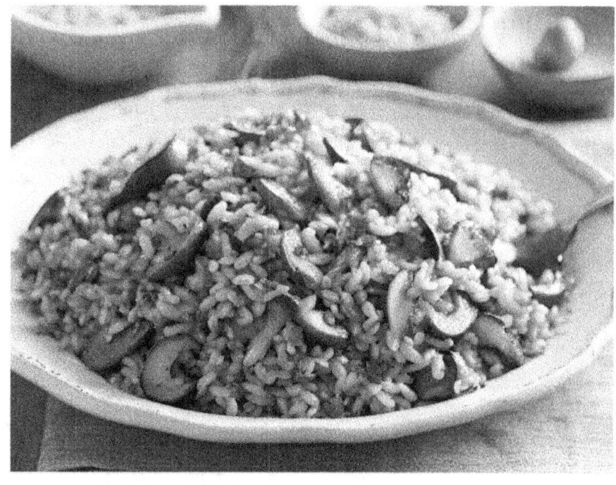

14. Garlic Roasted Potatoes

Ingredients:

- 2 pounds baby potatoes, halved
- 3 tablespoons olive oil
- 6 garlic cloves, minced
- 1 teaspoon dried rosemary
- 1 teaspoon dried thyme

Instructions:

1. Preheat the oven to 400°F (200°C). Line a baking sheet with parchment paper.
2. In a large bowl, toss the halved baby potatoes with olive oil, minced garlic, rosemary, and thyme until evenly coated.
3. Spread the potatoes in a single layer on the prepared baking sheet.
4. Roast in the preheated oven for 25-30 minutes, until the potatoes are golden and crispy on the edges.
5. Serve immediately.

Nutrition Info (per serving):

- Calories: 200
- Protein: 4g
- Carbohydrates: 34g
- Dietary Fiber: 5g
- Sugars: 2g
- Fat: 7g
- Saturated Fat: 1g
- Sodium: 20mg

Serves: 4 Cooking Time: 30 minutes

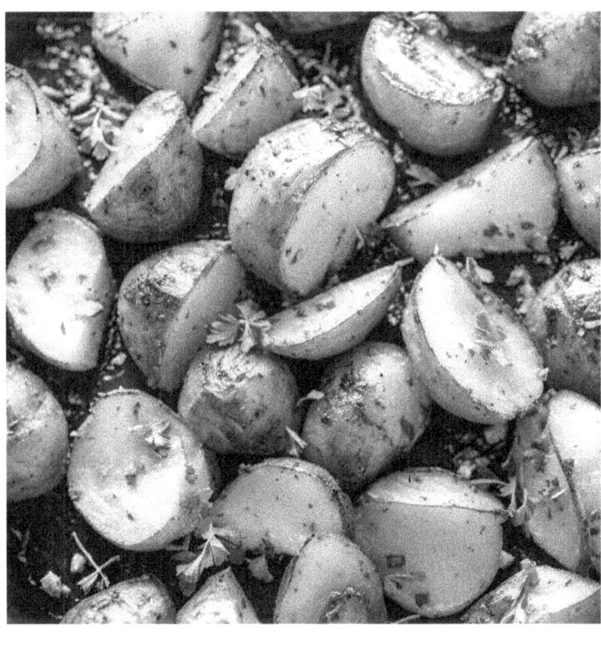

15. Bok Choy with Ginger Soy Sauce
Ingredients:
- 1 pound baby bok choy, halved lengthwise
- 2 tablespoons olive oil
- 2 garlic cloves, minced
- 1 tablespoon fresh ginger, grated
- 2 tablespoons low-sodium soy sauce
- 1 tablespoon rice vinegar
- 1 teaspoon honey
- 1 teaspoon sesame oil

Instructions:
1. Heat the olive oil in a large skillet over medium heat.
2. Add the minced garlic and grated ginger, and cook for 1-2 minutes until fragrant.
3. Add the halved bok choy, cut side down, and cook for 2-3 minutes until lightly browned.
4. In a small bowl, mix the soy sauce, rice vinegar, honey, and sesame oil.
5. Pour the sauce over the bok choy and cook for another 3-4 minutes until the bok choy is tender and the sauce has reduced slightly.
6. Serve immediately.

Nutrition Info (per serving):
- Calories: 100
- Protein: 3g
- Carbohydrates: 8g
- Dietary Fiber: 2g
- Sugars: 4g
- Fat: 7g
- Saturated Fat: 1g
- Sodium: 330mg

Serves: 4 Cooking Time: 15 minutes

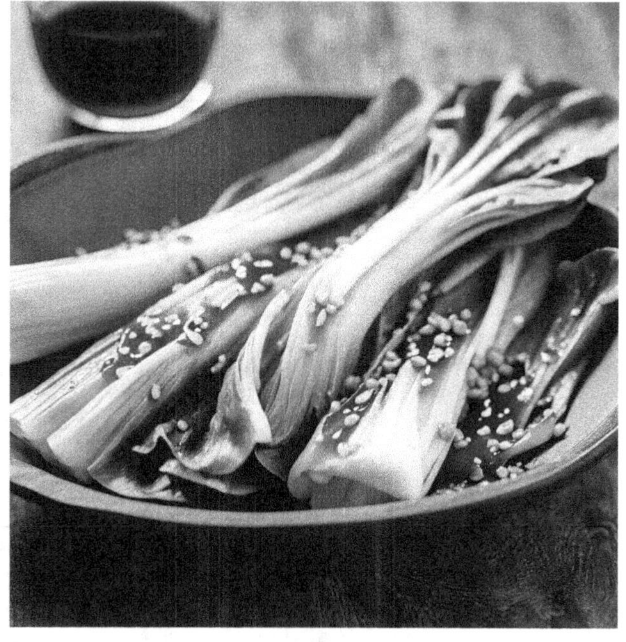

16. Kabocha Squash Curry

Ingredients:

- 1 kabocha squash, peeled, seeded, and cubed
- 2 tablespoons olive oil
- 1 large onion, chopped
- 3 garlic cloves, minced
- 1 tablespoon fresh ginger, grated
- 2 tablespoons curry powder
- 1 can (14 ounces) coconut milk (unsweetened)
- 1 cup low-sodium vegetable broth
- 1 cup diced tomatoes (canned or fresh)
- 1 cup chickpeas, cooked and drained
- 1/4 cup fresh cilantro, chopped

Instructions:

1. Heat the olive oil in a large pot over medium heat.
2. Add the chopped onion and cook until softened, about 5 minutes.
3. Add the minced garlic and grated ginger, and cook for another 1-2 minutes until fragrant.
4. Stir in the curry powder and cook for 1 minute.
5. Add the cubed kabocha squash, coconut milk, vegetable broth, and diced tomatoes. Bring to a simmer.
6. Cover and cook for 20-25 minutes, until the squash is tender.
7. Stir in the cooked chickpeas and cook for another 5 minutes until heated through.
8. Garnish with fresh cilantro before serving.
9. Serve immediately.

Nutrition Info (per serving):

- Calories: 280
- Protein: 6g
- Carbohydrates: 34g
- Dietary Fiber: 8g
- Sugars: 9g
- Fat: 14g
- Saturated Fat: 7g
- Sodium: 300mg

Serves: 4 Cooking Time: 40 minutes

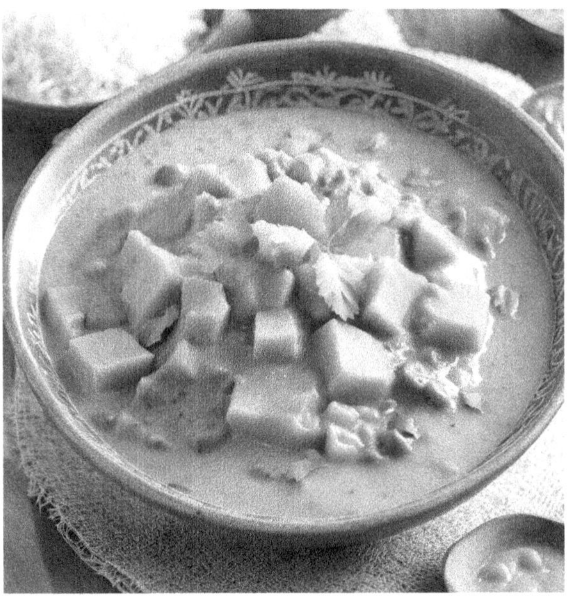

Soup & Stew Recipes

1. Lentil and Spinach Soup

Ingredients:

- 2 tablespoons olive oil
- 1 large onion, chopped
- 3 garlic cloves, minced
- 2 carrots, peeled and diced
- 2 celery stalks, diced
- 1 cup dried lentils, rinsed
- 1 can (14.5 ounces) diced tomatoes, with juice
- 6 cups low-sodium vegetable broth
- 1 teaspoon dried thyme
- 1 teaspoon cumin
- 4 cups fresh spinach, chopped
- 1 tablespoon lemon juice

Instructions:

1. Heat the olive oil in a large pot over medium heat.
2. Add the chopped onion, carrots, and celery, and cook until softened, about 5 minutes.
3. Add the minced garlic and cook for another 1-2 minutes until fragrant.
4. Stir in the lentils, diced tomatoes, vegetable broth, thyme, and cumin. Bring to a boil.
5. Reduce the heat and simmer for 25-30 minutes, until the lentils are tender.
6. Stir in the chopped spinach and cook for another 5 minutes until wilted.
7. Add the lemon juice and stir well.
8. Serve immediately.

Nutrition Info (per serving):

- Calories: 220
- Protein: 10g
- Carbohydrates: 34g
- Dietary Fiber: 12g
- Sugars: 7g
- Fat: 6g
- Saturated Fat: 1g
- Sodium: 150mg

Serves: 6 Cooking Time: 40 minutes

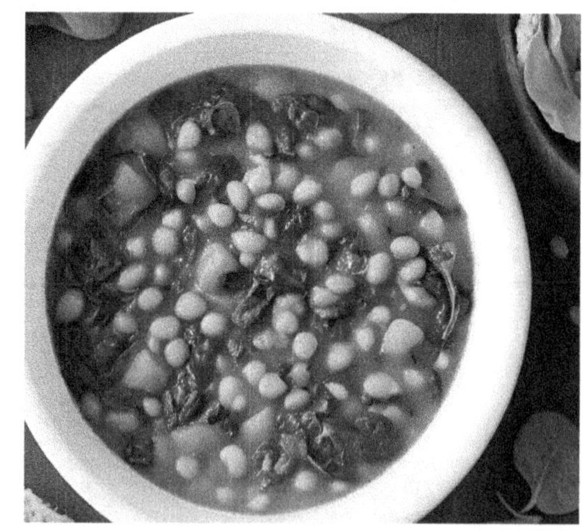

2. Beef and Barley Soup

Ingredients:

- 1 pound lean beef stew meat, cut into bite-sized pieces
- 2 tablespoons olive oil
- 1 large onion, chopped
- 3 garlic cloves, minced
- 2 carrots, peeled and diced
- 2 celery stalks, diced
- 1 cup pearl barley
- 6 cups low-sodium beef broth
- 1 can (14.5 ounces) diced tomatoes, with juice
- 1 teaspoon dried thyme
- 1 bay leaf
- 1 cup mushrooms, sliced

Instructions:

1. Heat the olive oil in a large pot over medium-high heat.
2. Add the beef stew meat and cook until browned on all sides. Remove the beef and set aside.
3. In the same pot, add the chopped onion, carrots, and celery, and cook until softened, about 5 minutes.
4. Add the minced garlic and cook for another 1-2 minutes.
5. Stir in the pearl barley, beef broth, diced tomatoes, thyme, and bay leaf. Return the beef to the pot.
6. Bring to a boil, then reduce the heat and simmer for 45-50 minutes, until the barley is tender.
7. Add the sliced mushrooms and cook for another 10 minutes.
8. Remove the bay leaf before serving.
9. Serve immediately.

Nutrition Info (per serving):

- Calories: 310
- Protein: 20g
- Carbohydrates: 34g
- Dietary Fiber: 8g
- Sugars: 6g
- Fat: 10g
- Saturated Fat: 2g
- Sodium: 300mg

Serves: 6 Cooking Time: 1 hour

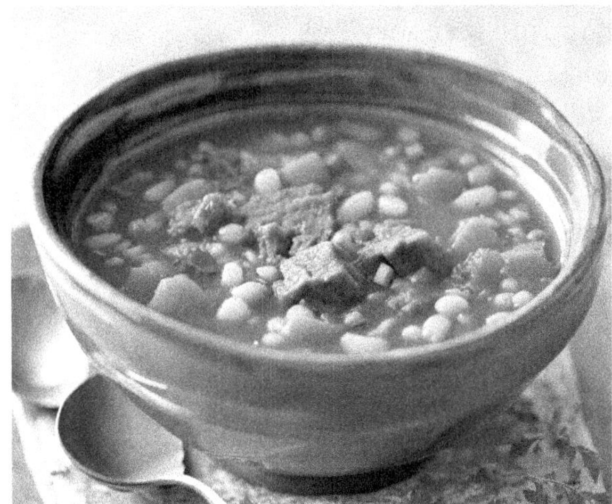

3. Vegetable Beef Stew

Ingredients:

- 1 pound lean beef stew meat, cut into bite-sized pieces
- 2 tablespoons olive oil
- 1 large onion, chopped
- 3 garlic cloves, minced
- 2 carrots, peeled and diced
- 2 celery stalks, diced
- 2 potatoes, peeled and diced
- 1 cup green beans, trimmed and cut into 1-inch pieces
- 1 can (14.5 ounces) diced tomatoes, with juice
- 6 cups low-sodium beef broth
- 1 teaspoon dried thyme
- 1 teaspoon dried rosemary
- 1 bay leaf

Instructions:

1. Heat the olive oil in a large pot over medium-high heat.
2. Add the beef stew meat and cook until browned on all sides. Remove the beef and set aside.
3. In the same pot, add the chopped onion, carrots, and celery, and cook until softened, about 5 minutes.
4. Add the minced garlic and cook for another 1-2 minutes.
5. Stir in the potatoes, green beans, diced tomatoes, beef broth, thyme, rosemary, and bay leaf. Return the beef to the pot.
6. Bring to a boil, then reduce the heat and simmer for 45-50 minutes, until the vegetables are tender.
7. Remove the bay leaf before serving.
8. Serve immediately.

Nutrition Info (per serving):

- Calories: 320
- Protein: 22g
- Carbohydrates: 28g
- Dietary Fiber: 6g
- Sugars: 6g
- Fat: 12g
- Saturated Fat: 3g
- Sodium: 300mg

Serves: 6 Cooking Time: 1 hour

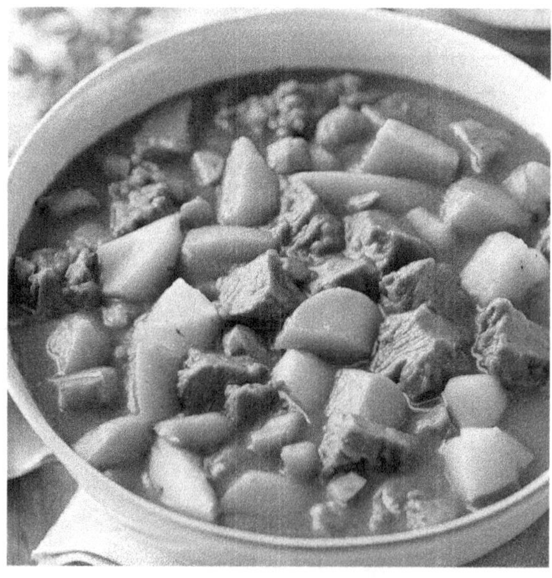

4. Split Pea Soup with Ham

Ingredients:

- 1 tablespoon olive oil
- 1 large onion, chopped
- 3 garlic cloves, minced
- 2 carrots, peeled and diced
- 2 celery stalks, diced
- 1 pound dried split peas, rinsed
- 1 meaty ham bone or 2 cups diced ham
- 6 cups low-sodium chicken broth
- 1 bay leaf
- 1 teaspoon dried thyme

Instructions:

1. Heat the olive oil in a large pot over medium heat.
2. Add the chopped onion, carrots, and celery, and cook until softened, about 5 minutes.
3. Add the minced garlic and cook for another 1-2 minutes.
4. Stir in the split peas, ham bone or diced ham, chicken broth, bay leaf, and thyme. Bring to a boil.
5. Reduce the heat and simmer for 1 hour, until the peas are tender.
6. Remove the ham bone and bay leaf. If using a ham bone, remove the meat from the bone, chop it, and return it to the soup.
7. Use an immersion blender to partially puree the soup for a thicker consistency, if desired.
8. Serve immediately.

Nutrition Info (per serving):

- Calories: 280
- Protein: 20g
- Carbohydrates: 40g
- Dietary Fiber: 16g
- Sugars: 8g
- Fat: 6g
- Saturated Fat: 1.5g
- Sodium: 350mg

Serves: 6 Cooking Time: 1 hour 10 minutes

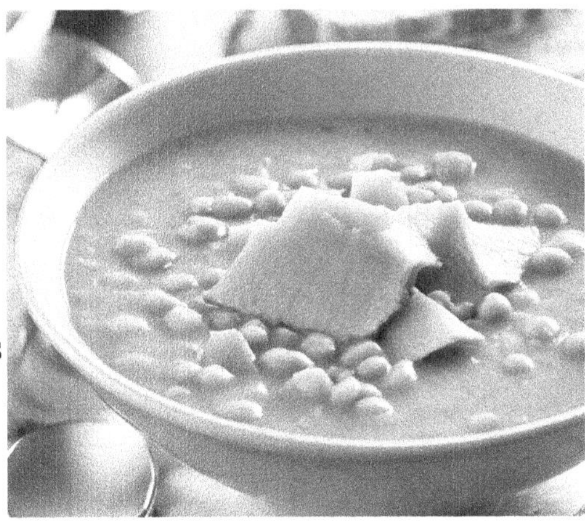

5. Italian White Bean and Kale Soup
Ingredients:
- 2 tablespoons olive oil
- 1 large onion, chopped
- 3 garlic cloves, minced
- 2 carrots, peeled and diced
- 2 celery stalks, diced
- 6 cups low-sodium vegetable broth
- 1 can (14.5 ounces) diced tomatoes, with juice
- 2 cans (15 ounces each) white beans, rinsed and drained
- 1 teaspoon dried oregano
- 1 teaspoon dried basil
- 4 cups kale, chopped
- 1 tablespoon lemon juice

Instructions:
1. Heat the olive oil in a large pot over medium heat.
2. Add the chopped onion, carrots, and celery, and cook until softened, about 5 minutes.
3. Add the minced garlic and cook for another 1-2 minutes.
4. Stir in the vegetable broth, diced tomatoes, white beans, oregano, and basil. Bring to a boil.
5. Reduce the heat and simmer for 20 minutes.
6. Add the chopped kale and cook for another 5 minutes until wilted.
7. Stir in the lemon juice and serve immediately.

Nutrition Info (per serving):
- Calories: 200
- Protein: 8g
- Carbohydrates: 32g
- Dietary Fiber: 9g
- Sugars: 7g
- Fat: 6g
- Saturated Fat: 1g
- Sodium: 300mg

Serves: 6 Cooking Time: 30 minutes

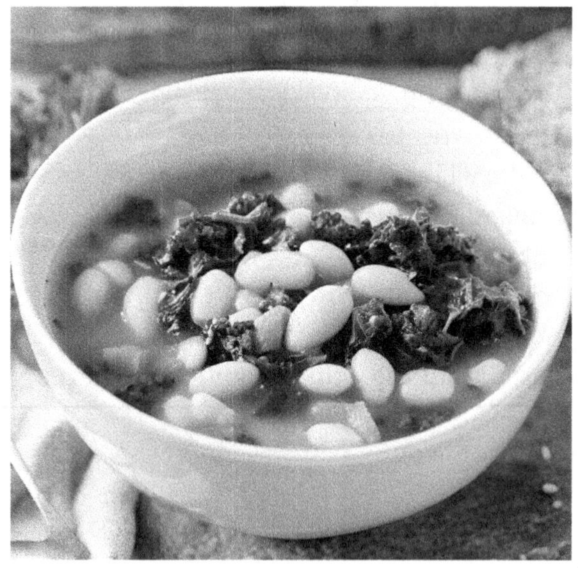

6. Turkey and Wild Rice Soup

Ingredients:

- 2 tablespoons olive oil
- 1 large onion, chopped
- 3 garlic cloves, minced
- 2 carrots, peeled and diced
- 2 celery stalks, diced
- 1 cup wild rice, rinsed
- 6 cups low-sodium chicken broth
- 2 cups cooked turkey, shredded
- 1 teaspoon dried thyme
- 1 bay leaf
- 1 cup unsweetened almond milk
- 2 tablespoons fresh parsley, chopped

Instructions:

1. Heat the olive oil in a large pot over medium heat.
2. Add the chopped onion, carrots, and celery, and cook until softened, about 5 minutes.
3. Add the minced garlic and cook for another 1-2 minutes.
4. Stir in the wild rice, chicken broth, shredded turkey, thyme, and bay leaf. Bring to a boil.
5. Reduce the heat and simmer for 40-45 minutes, until the rice is tender.
6. Stir in the almond milk and cook for another 5 minutes.
7. Remove the bay leaf and garnish with fresh parsley before serving.

Nutrition Info (per serving):

- Calories: 250
- Protein: 18g
- Carbohydrates: 28g
- Dietary Fiber: 4g
- Sugars: 4g
- Fat: 9g
- Saturated Fat: 1.5g
- Sodium: 300mg

Serves: 6 Cooking Time: 50 minutes

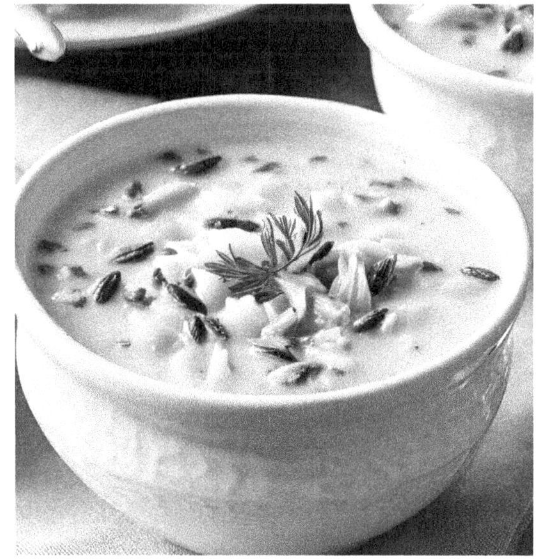

7. Mushroom and Thyme Soup

Ingredients:

- 2 tablespoons olive oil
- 1 large onion, chopped
- 3 garlic cloves, minced
- 1 pound mushrooms, sliced
- 6 cups low-sodium vegetable broth
- 1 cup unsweetened almond milk
- 1 teaspoon dried thyme
- 1 bay leaf
- 1 tablespoon fresh parsley, chopped

Instructions:

1. Heat the olive oil in a large pot over medium heat.
2. Add the chopped onion and cook until softened, about 5 minutes.
3. Add the minced garlic and sliced mushrooms, and cook until the mushrooms are tender, about 5-7 minutes.
4. Stir in the vegetable broth, almond milk, thyme, and bay leaf. Bring to a boil.
5. Reduce the heat and simmer for 20 minutes.
6. Remove the bay leaf and garnish with fresh parsley before serving.
7. Serve immediately.

Nutrition Info (per serving):

- Calories: 140
- Protein: 5g
- Carbohydrates: 12g
- Dietary Fiber: 3g
- Sugars: 4g
- Fat: 9g
- Saturated Fat: 1.5g
- Sodium: 250mg

Serves: 6 Cooking Time: 30 minutes

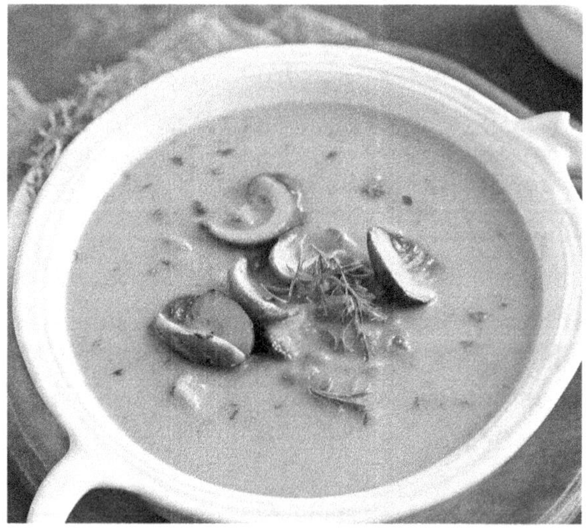

8. Beetroot and Cabbage Borscht

Ingredients:

- 2 tablespoons olive oil
- 1 large onion, chopped
- 3 garlic cloves, minced
- 2 carrots, peeled and grated
- 2 beets, peeled and grated
- 1/2 head of cabbage, thinly sliced
- 6 cups low-sodium vegetable broth
- 1 can (14.5 ounces) diced tomatoes, with juice
- 1 bay leaf
- 1 tablespoon apple cider vinegar
- 1 tablespoon honey
- 1/4 cup fresh dill, chopped
- 1/2 cup plain Greek yogurt (optional, for garnish)

Instructions:

1. Heat the olive oil in a large pot over medium heat.
2. Add the chopped onion and cook until softened, about 5 minutes.
3. Add the minced garlic, grated carrots, and grated beets, and cook for another 5 minutes.
4. Stir in the vegetable broth, diced tomatoes, sliced cabbage, and bay leaf. Bring to a boil.
5. Reduce the heat and simmer for 30 minutes, until the vegetables are tender.
6. Stir in the apple cider vinegar and honey.
7. Remove the bay leaf and garnish with fresh dill.
8. Serve with a dollop of plain Greek yogurt if desired.

Nutrition Info (per serving):

- Calories: 180
- Protein: 4g
- Carbohydrates: 28g
- Dietary Fiber: 7g
- Sugars: 15g
- Fat: 6g
- Saturated Fat: 1g
- Sodium: 260mg

Serves: 6 Cooking Time: 45 minutes

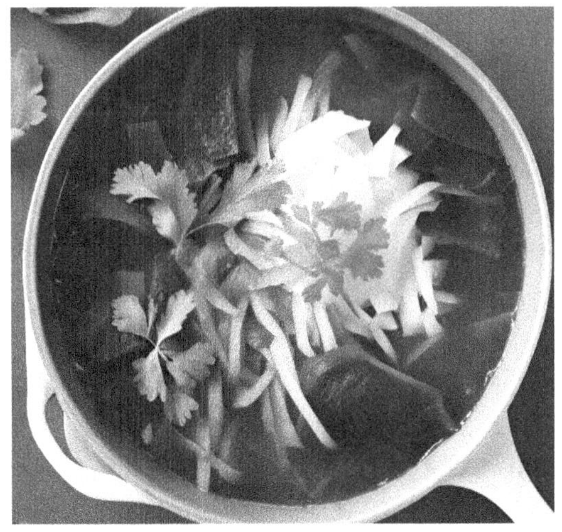

9. Thai Coconut Chicken Soup (Tom Kha Gai)

Ingredients:

- 1 tablespoon olive oil
- 1 onion, chopped
- 3 garlic cloves, minced
- 1 tablespoon fresh ginger, grated
- 1 stalk lemongrass, cut into 3-inch pieces and bruised
- 3 cups low-sodium chicken broth
- 1 can (14 ounces) coconut milk (unsweetened)
- 1 pound boneless, skinless chicken breasts, thinly sliced
- 1 cup mushrooms, sliced
- 1 red bell pepper, thinly sliced
- 3 tablespoons fish sauce
- 1 tablespoon lime juice
- 1 teaspoon turmeric
- 1/4 cup fresh cilantro, chopped

Instructions:

1. Heat the olive oil in a large pot over medium heat.
2. Add the chopped onion, minced garlic, and grated ginger, and cook until fragrant, about 2-3 minutes.
3. Add the lemongrass pieces and cook for another 1-2 minutes.
4. Pour in the chicken broth and bring to a boil. Reduce the heat and simmer for 10 minutes.
5. Add the coconut milk, chicken slices, mushrooms, and red bell pepper. Simmer for another 10 minutes until the chicken is cooked through.
6. Stir in the fish sauce, lime juice, and turmeric. Cook for an additional 2-3 minutes.
7. Remove the lemongrass pieces before serving.
8. Garnish with fresh cilantro and serve immediately.

Nutrition Info (per serving):

- Calories: 270
- Protein: 22g
- Carbohydrates: 10g
- Dietary Fiber: 2g
- Sugars: 3g
- Fat: 17g
- Saturated Fat: 12g
- Sodium: 550mg

Serves: 4 Cooking Time: 30 minutes

10. Fisherman's Soup with Tomato and Saffron

Ingredients:

- 2 tablespoons olive oil
- 1 large onion, chopped
- 3 garlic cloves, minced
- 1 fennel bulb, thinly sliced
- 1 can (14.5 ounces) diced tomatoes, with juice
- 4 cups low-sodium fish or vegetable broth
- 1/4 teaspoon saffron threads
- 1 pound firm white fish (such as cod or halibut), cut into chunks
- 1/2 pound shrimp, peeled and deveined
- 1/4 cup fresh parsley, chopped
- 1 tablespoon lemon juice

Instructions:

1. Heat the olive oil in a large pot over medium heat.
2. Add the chopped onion, minced garlic, and sliced fennel, and cook until softened, about 5 minutes.
3. Stir in the diced tomatoes with their juice, fish or vegetable broth, and saffron threads. Bring to a boil.
4. Reduce the heat and simmer for 15 minutes to allow the flavors to meld.
5. Add the fish chunks and shrimp, and simmer for another 5-7 minutes until the fish is opaque and the shrimp are pink and cooked through.
6. Stir in the fresh parsley and lemon juice.
7. Serve immediately.

Nutrition Info (per serving):

- Calories: 250
- Protein: 32g
- Carbohydrates: 12g
- Dietary Fiber: 3g
- Sugars: 6g
- Fat: 8g
- Saturated Fat: 1.5g
- Sodium: 450mg

Serves: 4 Cooking Time: 30 minutes

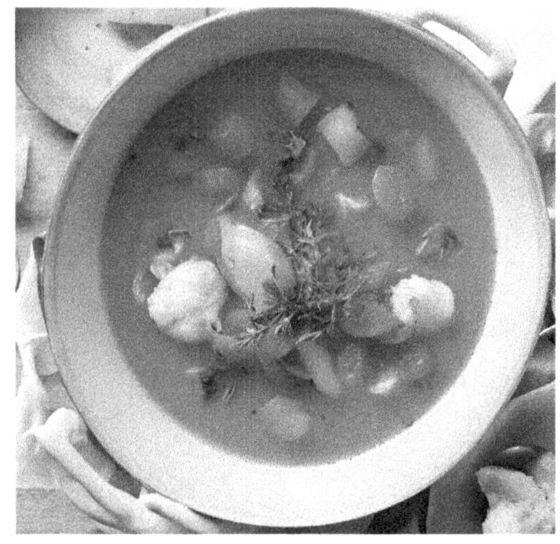

11. Sweet Potato and Black Bean Chili

Ingredients:

- 2 tablespoons olive oil
- 1 large onion, chopped
- 3 garlic cloves, minced
- 2 sweet potatoes, peeled and diced
- 1 red bell pepper, chopped
- 1 yellow bell pepper, chopped
- 1 can (14.5 ounces) diced tomatoes, with juice
- 2 cans (15 ounces each) black beans, rinsed and drained
- 4 cups low-sodium vegetable broth
- 1 tablespoon chili powder
- 1 teaspoon ground cumin
- 1 teaspoon smoked paprika
- 1/4 teaspoon cayenne pepper (optional)
- 1/4 cup fresh cilantro, chopped
- 1 avocado, diced (for garnish)

Instructions:

1. Heat the olive oil in a large pot over medium heat.
2. Add the chopped onion and cook until softened, about 5 minutes.
3. Add the minced garlic, diced sweet potatoes, and chopped bell peppers, and cook for another 5 minutes.
4. Stir in the diced tomatoes, black beans, vegetable broth, chili powder, ground cumin, smoked paprika, and cayenne pepper (if using). Bring to a boil.
5. Reduce the heat and simmer for 25-30 minutes, until the sweet potatoes are tender.
6. Stir in the chopped cilantro.
7. Serve the chili garnished with diced avocado.

Nutrition Info (per serving):

- Calories: 300
- Protein: 10g
- Carbohydrates: 50g
- Dietary Fiber: 12g
- Sugars: 12g
- Fat: 10g
- Saturated Fat: 1.5g
- Sodium: 450mg

Serves: 6 Cooking Time: 40 minutes

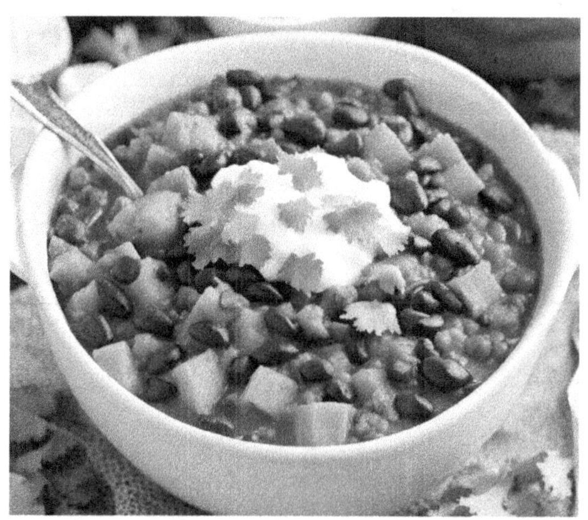

12. Pea and Ham Hock Soup

Ingredients:

- 1 tablespoon olive oil
- 1 large onion, chopped
- 3 garlic cloves, minced
- 2 carrots, peeled and diced
- 2 celery stalks, diced
- 1 pound dried split peas, rinsed
- 1 meaty ham hock
- 6 cups low-sodium chicken broth
- 1 bay leaf
- 1 teaspoon dried thyme
- 1/4 cup fresh parsley, chopped

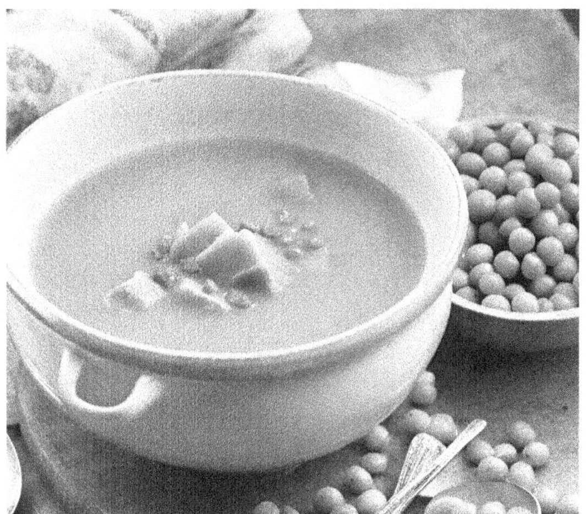

Instructions:

1. Heat the olive oil in a large pot over medium heat.
2. Add the chopped onion, carrots, and celery, and cook until softened, about 5 minutes.
3. Add the minced garlic and cook for another 1-2 minutes.
4. Stir in the split peas, ham hock, chicken broth, bay leaf, and thyme. Bring to a boil.
5. Reduce the heat and simmer for 1 hour, until the peas are tender.
6. Remove the ham hock and bay leaf. Shred the meat from the ham hock and return it to the soup.
7. Use an immersion blender to partially puree the soup for a thicker consistency, if desired.
8. Garnish with fresh parsley before serving.

Nutrition Info (per serving):

- Calories: 270
- Protein: 20g
- Carbohydrates: 35g
- Dietary Fiber: 14g
- Sugars: 8g
- Fat: 7g
- Saturated Fat: 2g
- Sodium: 350mg

Serves: 6 Cooking Time: 1 hour 15 minutes

13. Italian Sausage and Tortellini Soup

Ingredients:

- 1 tablespoon olive oil
- 1 pound Italian sausage (ensure it's low in sodium and free from nitrates)
- 1 large onion, chopped
- 3 garlic cloves, minced
- 2 carrots, peeled and sliced
- 2 celery stalks, sliced
- 6 cups low-sodium chicken broth
- 1 can (14.5 ounces) diced tomatoes, with juice
- 1 teaspoon dried basil
- 1 teaspoon dried oregano
- 1 package (9 ounces) cheese tortellini (ensure it's low in sodium)
- 4 cups fresh spinach, chopped
- 1/4 cup grated Parmesan cheese (optional)
- 1/4 cup fresh parsley, chopped

Instructions:

1. Heat the olive oil in a large pot over medium heat.
2. Add the Italian sausage, breaking it up with a spoon, and cook until browned. Remove the sausage from the pot and set aside.
3. In the same pot, add the chopped onion, carrots, and celery, and cook until softened, about 5 minutes.
4. Add the minced garlic and cook for another 1-2 minutes.
5. Stir in the chicken broth, diced tomatoes, basil, and oregano. Bring to a boil.
6. Return the sausage to the pot and reduce the heat. Simmer for 15 minutes.
7. Add the tortellini and cook according to package instructions, usually about 7-9 minutes.
8. Stir in the chopped spinach and cook for another 2-3 minutes until wilted.
9. Serve the soup garnished with grated Parmesan cheese and fresh parsley, if desired.

Nutrition Info (per serving):

- Calories: 350
- Protein: 20g
- Carbohydrates: 25g
- Dietary Fiber: 5g
- Sugars: 6g
- Fat: 18g
- Saturated Fat: 6g
- Sodium: 450mg

Serves: 6 Cooking Time: 35 minutes

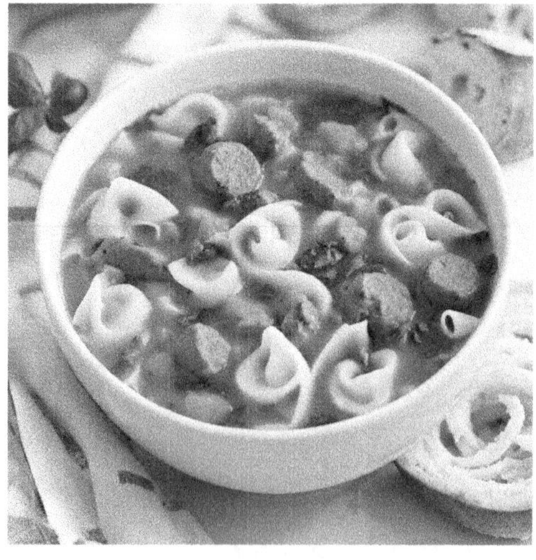

14. Winter Vegetable Stew

Ingredients:

- 2 tablespoons olive oil
- 1 large onion, chopped
- 3 garlic cloves, minced
- 2 carrots, peeled and chopped
- 2 parsnips, peeled and chopped
- 2 sweet potatoes, peeled and chopped
- 1 turnip, peeled and chopped
- 1 can (14.5 ounces) diced tomatoes, with juice
- 6 cups low-sodium vegetable broth
- 1 teaspoon dried thyme
- 1 teaspoon dried rosemary
- 1/2 teaspoon cumin
- 1/4 teaspoon cayenne pepper (optional)
- 1/4 cup fresh parsley, chopped

Instructions:

1. Heat the olive oil in a large pot over medium heat.
2. Add the chopped onion and cook until softened, about 5 minutes.
3. Add the minced garlic and cook for another 1-2 minutes.
4. Stir in the carrots, parsnips, sweet potatoes, and turnip. Cook for 5 minutes.
5. Add the diced tomatoes, vegetable broth, thyme, rosemary, cumin, and cayenne pepper (if using). Bring to a boil.
6. Reduce the heat and simmer for 30 minutes, until the vegetables are tender.
7. Stir in the fresh parsley before serving.
8. Serve immediately.

Nutrition Info (per serving):

- Calories: 220
- Protein: 4g
- Carbohydrates: 40g
- Dietary Fiber: 8g
- Sugars: 12g
- Fat: 7g
- Saturated Fat: 1g
- Sodium: 300mg

Serves: 6 Cooking Time: 40 minutes

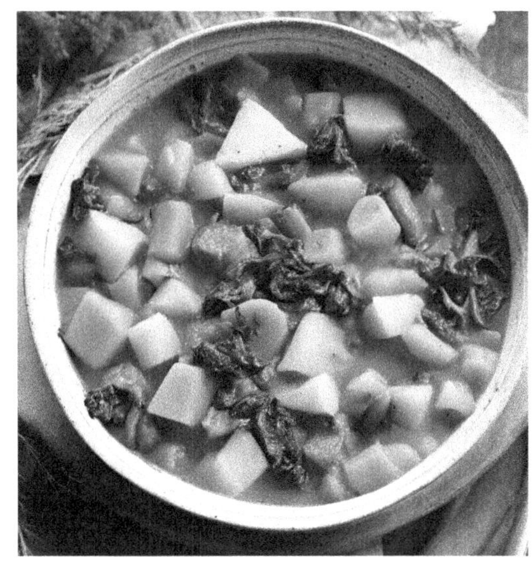

15. Spiced Chickpea Stew

Ingredients:

- 2 tablespoons olive oil
- 1 large onion, chopped
- 3 garlic cloves, minced
- 1 tablespoon fresh ginger, grated
- 2 carrots, peeled and chopped
- 1 sweet potato, peeled and chopped
- 1 red bell pepper, chopped
- 1 can (14.5 ounces) diced tomatoes, with juice
- 4 cups low-sodium vegetable broth
- 2 cans (15 ounces each) chickpeas, rinsed and drained
- 1 teaspoon ground cumin
- 1 teaspoon ground coriander
- 1/2 teaspoon ground turmeric
- 1/4 teaspoon cayenne pepper (optional)
- 1/4 cup fresh cilantro, chopped

Instructions:

1. Heat the olive oil in a large pot over medium heat.
2. Add the chopped onion and cook until softened, about 5 minutes.
3. Add the minced garlic and grated ginger, and cook for another 1-2 minutes.
4. Stir in the carrots, sweet potato, and red bell pepper. Cook for 5 minutes.
5. Add the diced tomatoes, vegetable broth, chickpeas, cumin, coriander, turmeric, and cayenne pepper (if using). Bring to a boil.
6. Reduce the heat and simmer for 25-30 minutes, until the vegetables are tender.
7. Stir in the fresh cilantro before serving.
8. Serve immediately.

Nutrition Info (per serving):

- Calories: 260
- Protein: 8g
- Carbohydrates: 42g
- Dietary Fiber: 10g
- Sugars: 10g
- Fat: 8g
- Saturated Fat: 1g
- Sodium: 350mg

Serves: 6 Cooking Time: 35 minutes

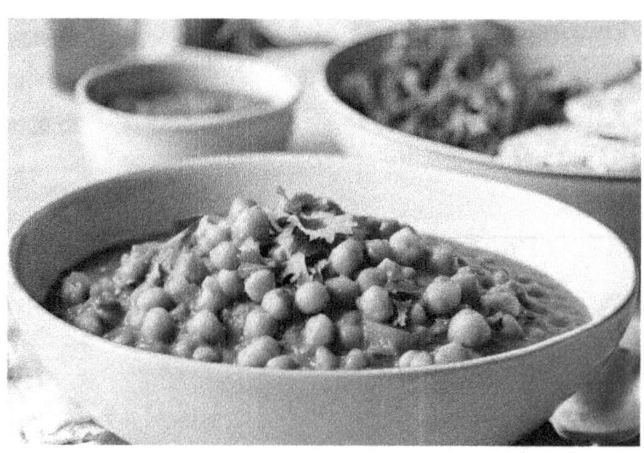

16. Russian Mushroom and Potato Soup

Ingredients:

- 2 tablespoons olive oil
- 1 large onion, chopped
- 3 garlic cloves, minced
- 1 pound mushrooms, sliced
- 3 potatoes, peeled and diced
- 6 cups low-sodium vegetable broth
- 1 teaspoon dried dill
- 1/2 teaspoon paprika
- 1 bay leaf
- 1/4 cup fresh dill, chopped
- 1/2 cup plain Greek yogurt (optional, for garnish)

Instructions:

1. Heat the olive oil in a large pot over medium heat.
2. Add the chopped onion and cook until softened, about 5 minutes.
3. Add the minced garlic and sliced mushrooms, and cook until the mushrooms are tender, about 5-7 minutes.
4. Stir in the diced potatoes, vegetable broth, dried dill, paprika, and bay leaf. Bring to a boil.
5. Reduce the heat and simmer for 20-25 minutes, until the potatoes are tender.
6. Remove the bay leaf and stir in the fresh dill.
7. Serve the soup with a dollop of plain Greek yogurt, if desired.

Nutrition Info (per serving):

- Calories: 200
- Protein: 6g
- Carbohydrates: 30g
- Dietary Fiber: 5g
- Sugars: 5g
- Fat: 7g
- Saturated Fat: 1.5g
- Sodium: 250mg

Serves: 6 Cooking Time: 35 minutes

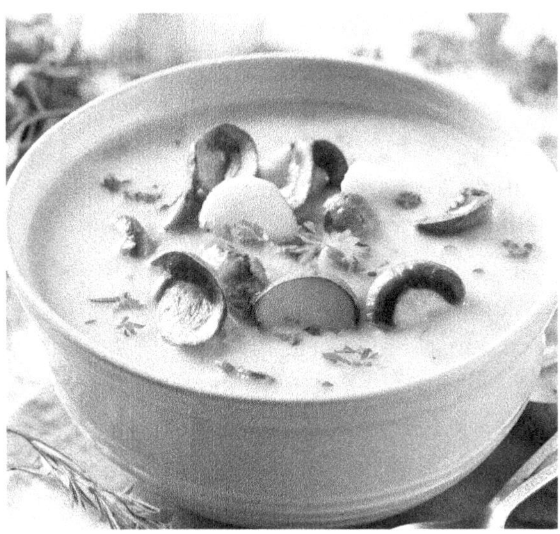

10-WEEK MEAL PLAN

Week 1
Monday
- Breakfast: Blueberry Almond Smoothie
- Lunch: Chicken Salad with Avocado
- Dinner: Lemon Herb Roasted Chicken with Roasted Brussels Sprouts with Balsamic Glaze
- Snack: Greek Yogurt with Mixed Berries

Tuesday
- Breakfast: Berry Beet Smoothie
- Lunch: Lentil and Spinach Soup
- Dinner: Grilled Turkey Burgers with Sauteed Green Beans with Garlic
- Snack: Hummus and Cucumber Sandwich

Wednesday
- Breakfast: Oatmeal with Walnuts and Berries
- Lunch: Spaghetti Squash with Tomato Sauce
- Dinner: Herb Roasted Chicken Thighs with Butternut Squash Risotto
- Snack: Fruit Salad with Mint

Thursday
- Breakfast: Creamy Buckwheat Porridge
- Lunch: Winter Vegetable Stew
- Dinner: Baked Salmon with Dill and Lemon with Steamed Vegetable Medley
- Snack: Kefir with Honey and Almonds

Friday
- Breakfast: Millet Porridge with Honey and Nuts
- Lunch: Mushroom and Barley Pilaf
- Dinner: Moroccan Turkey Stew
- Snack: Avocado Toast with Sesame Seeds

Saturday
- Breakfast: Soft Scrambled Eggs
- Lunch: Broccoli and Cashew Stir-Fry
- Dinner: Beef and Barley Soup
- Snack: Cottage Cheese Pancakes

Sunday
- Breakfast: Egg White Omelette with Spinach
- Lunch: Roasted Chicken with Squash and Cranberries
- Dinner: Poached Cod in Tomato Broth
- Snack: Melon and Prosciutto Plate

Week 2

Monday
- Breakfast: Silken Tofu Scramble
- Lunch: Vegetable Beef Stew
- Dinner: Ginger Soy Marinated Tuna with Sautéed Mushrooms
- Snack: Yogurt Parfait with Muesli

Tuesday
- Breakfast: Poached Eggs over Asparagus
- Lunch: Chicken Pho
- Dinner: Pistachio-Crusted Salmon with Carrot Ginger Soup
- Snack: Banana Oat Pancakes

Wednesday
- Breakfast: Greek Yogurt with Mixed Berries
- Lunch: Beet and Goat Cheese Salad
- Dinner: Turkey and Quinoa Stuffed Peppers
- Snack: Coconut Yogurt and Mango

Thursday
- Breakfast: Blueberry Almond Smoothie
- Lunch: Italian White Bean and Kale Soup
- Dinner: Herb-Crusted Tilapia with Spiced Sweet Potato Wedges
- Snack: Almond Flour Waffles

Friday
- Breakfast: Berry Beet Smoothie
- Lunch: Soft Scrambled Eggs
- Dinner: Balsamic Glazed Turkey Drumsticks with Sautéed Green Beans with Garlic
- Snack: Spiced Sweet Potato Wedges

Saturday
- Breakfast: Oatmeal with Walnuts and Berries
- Lunch: Mushroom and Thyme Soup
- Dinner: Mackerel Pate with Garlic Roasted Potatoes
- Snack: Avocado Toast with Sesame Seeds

Sunday
- Breakfast: Creamy Buckwheat Porridge
- Lunch: Chicken Cacciatore
- Dinner: Salmon Berry Salad
- Snack: Hummus and Cucumber Sandwich

Week 3

Monday

- Breakfast: Millet Porridge with Honey and Nuts
- Lunch: Roasted Chicken with Squash and Cranberries
- Dinner: Split Pea Soup with Ham
- Snack: Cottage Cheese Pancakes

Tuesday

- Breakfast: Soft Scrambled Eggs
- Lunch: Bok Choy with Ginger Soy Sauce
- Dinner: Lemon Garlic Tilapia with Mushroom and Barley Pilaf
- Snack: Kefir with Honey and Almonds

Wednesday

- Breakfast: Egg White Omelette with Spinach
- Lunch: Thai Coconut Chicken Soup (Tom Kha Gai)
- Dinner: Moroccan Spiced Salmon with Creamed Spinach
- Snack: Greek Yogurt with Mixed Berries

Thursday

- Breakfast: Silken Tofu Scramble
- Lunch: Turkey Chili
- Dinner: Shrimp and Quinoa Salad with Spiced Sweet Potato Wedges
- Snack: Melon and Prosciutto Plate

Friday

- Breakfast: Poached Eggs over Asparagus
- Lunch: Sweet Potato and Black Bean Chili
- Dinner: Trout Almondine with Sauteed Green Beans with Garlic
- Snack: Coconut Yogurt and Mango

Saturday

- Breakfast: Greek Yogurt with Mixed Berries
- Lunch: Chicken Salad with Avocado
- Dinner: Fisherman's Soup with Tomato and Saffron
- Snack: Yogurt Parfait with Muesli

Sunday

- Breakfast: Blueberry Almond Smoothie
- Lunch: Spiced Chickpea Stew
- Dinner: Herb Roasted Chicken Thighs with Steamed Vegetable Medley
- Snack: Avocado Toast with Sesame Seeds

Week 4
Monday

- Breakfast: Berry Beet Smoothie
- Lunch: Italian Sausage and Tortellini Soup
- Dinner: Haddock in Parchment with Vegetables and Roasted Brussels Sprouts with Balsamic Glaze
- Snack: Banana Oat Pancakes

Tuesday

- Breakfast: Oatmeal with Walnuts and Berries
- Lunch: Russian Mushroom and Potato Soup
- Dinner: Poached Cod in Tomato Broth
- Snack: Almond Flour Waffles

Wednesday

- Breakfast: Creamy Buckwheat Porridge
- Lunch: Roasted Chicken with Squash and Cranberries
- Dinner: Sea Bass with Fennel and Orange with Garlic Roasted Potatoes
- Snack: Fruit Salad with Mint

Thursday

- Breakfast: Millet Porridge with Honey and Nuts
- Lunch: Mushroom and Barley Pilaf
- Dinner: Herb-Crusted Tilapia with Spiced Sweet Potato Wedges
- Snack: Cottage Cheese Pancakes

Friday

- Breakfast: Soft Scrambled Eggs
- Lunch: Spaghetti Squash with Tomato Sauce
- Dinner: Beef and Barley Soup
- Snack: Hummus and Cucumber Sandwich

Saturday

- Breakfast: Egg White Omelette with Spinach
- Lunch: Vegetable Beef Stew
- Dinner: Shrimp Gazpacho with Sautéed Mushrooms
- Snack: Greek Yogurt with Mixed Berries

Sunday

- Breakfast: Silken Tofu Scramble
- Lunch: Chicken Pho
- Dinner: Roasted Chicken with Squash and Cranberries
- Snack: Melon and Prosciutto Plate

Week 5

Monday

- Breakfast: Poached Eggs over Asparagus
- Lunch: Chicken and Broccoli Stir-Fry
- Dinner: Baked Trout with Herb Butter and Roasted Brussels Sprouts with Balsamic Glaze
- Snack: Fruit Salad with Mint

Tuesday

- Breakfast: Greek Yogurt with Mixed Berries
- Lunch: Chicken Ginger Soup
- Dinner: Cod with Parsley Pesto and Garlic Roasted Potatoes
- Snack: Kefir with Honey and Almonds

Wednesday

- Breakfast: Blueberry Almond Smoothie
- Lunch: Sweet Potato and Black Bean Chili
- Dinner: Turkey Piccata with Steamed Vegetable Medley
- Snack: Yogurt Parfait with Muesli

Thursday

- Breakfast: Berry Beet Smoothie
- Lunch: Winter Vegetable Stew
- Dinner: Salmon Quiche with Dill and Spiced Sweet Potato Wedges
- Snack: Cottage Cheese Pancakes

Friday

- Breakfast: Oatmeal with Walnuts and Berries
- Lunch: Bok Choy with Ginger Soy Sauce
- Dinner: Mackerel Pate with Garlic Roasted Potatoes
- Snack: Coconut Yogurt and Mango

Saturday

- Breakfast: Creamy Buckwheat Porridge
- Lunch: Italian White Bean and Kale Soup
- Dinner: Smoked Turkey Breast with Spiced Sweet Potato Wedges
- Snack: Hummus and Cucumber Sandwich

Sunday

- Breakfast: Millet Porridge with Honey and Nuts
- Lunch: Mushroom and Thyme Soup
- Dinner: Baked Salmon with Dill and Lemon with Steamed Vegetable Medley
- Snack: Almond Flour Waffles

Week 6

Monday
- Breakfast: Buckwheat Pancakes with Honey
- Lunch: Mushroom and Cashew Stir-Fry
- Dinner: Peppercorn Tuna Steaks with Green Bean Almondine
- Snack: Greek Yogurt with Flaxseed and Blueberries

Tuesday
- Breakfast: Berry Chia Pudding
- Lunch: Cauliflower Steak with Herb Sauce
- Dinner: Grilled Swordfish with Mango Salsa
- Snack: Apple Slices with Almond Butter

Wednesday
- Breakfast: Banana Oatmeal with Chia Seeds
- Lunch: Lentil and Quinoa Salad with Lemon Dressing
- Dinner: Baked Cod with Panko Crust and Steamed Asparagus
- Snack: Trail Mix with Nuts and Dried Fruits

Thursday
- Breakfast: Pumpkin Smoothie with Cinnamon
- Lunch: Spiced Chickpea and Kale Soup
- Dinner: Sesame Crusted Salmon with Stir-Fried Bok Choy
- Snack: Hummus with Carrot and Celery Sticks

Friday
- Breakfast: Spinach and Feta Omelette
- Lunch: Sweet Potato and Black Bean Tacos
- Dinner: Ginger Soy Glazed Scallops with Quinoa Pilaf
- Snack: Fresh Pineapple Slices

Saturday
- Breakfast: Almond Butter Toast with Banana Slices
- Lunch: Roasted Beet and Goat Cheese Salad
- Dinner: Chicken Satay with Peanut Sauce and Cucumber Salad
- Snack: Cucumber and Avocado Rolls

Sunday
- Breakfast: Berry and Spinach Smoothie
- Lunch: Spaghetti Squash Primavera
- Dinner: Herb Marinated Grilled Shrimp with Brown Rice
- Snack: Baked Apple Chips

Week 7

Monday

- Breakfast: Vanilla Almond Overnight Oats
- Lunch: Cucumber and Avocado Sushi Rolls
- Dinner: Lemon Dill Baked Haddock with Broccoli
- Snack: Greek Yogurt with Honey and Walnuts

Tuesday

- Breakfast: Berry and Flaxseed Smoothie
- Lunch: Zucchini Noodles with Pesto and Cherry Tomatoes
- Dinner: Grilled Halibut with Roasted Brussels Sprouts
- Snack: Roasted Chickpeas

Wednesday

- Breakfast: Apple Cinnamon Quinoa
- Lunch: Butternut Squash Soup with Pumpkin Seeds
- Dinner: Baked Sole with Lemon Butter and Steamed Green Beans
- Snack: Pear Slices with Cottage Cheese

Thursday

- Breakfast: Peach and Almond Smoothie
- Lunch: Chickpea and Avocado Salad
- Dinner: Grilled Tilapia with Mango Avocado Salsa
- Snack: Celery Sticks with Hummus

Friday

- Breakfast: Avocado and Spinach Smoothie
- Lunch: Tomato Basil Soup with Whole Grain Bread
- Dinner: Blackened Mahi Mahi with Coconut Rice
- Snack: Mixed Berry Salad

Saturday

- Breakfast: Strawberry Banana Oatmeal
- Lunch: Grilled Vegetable Salad with Balsamic Dressing
- Dinner: Teriyaki Salmon with Brown Rice
- Snack: Fresh Orange Slices

Sunday

- Breakfast: Mixed Berry Parfait with Granola
- Lunch: Lentil and Vegetable Stew
- Dinner: Lemon Garlic Shrimp with Quinoa
- Snack: Edamame

Week 8

Monday

- Breakfast: Pineapple and Coconut Smoothie
- Lunch: Roasted Red Pepper and Tomato Soup
- Dinner: Garlic and Herb Baked Chicken with Asparagus
- Snack: Carrot Sticks with Tzatziki

Tuesday

- Breakfast: Cherry Almond Overnight Oats
- Lunch: Spinach and Strawberry Salad with Balsamic Vinaigrette
- Dinner: Grilled Swordfish with Lemon Butter
- Snack: Apple Slices with Almond Butter

Wednesday

- Breakfast: Peach and Chia Seed Pudding
- Lunch: Quinoa and Black Bean Salad
- Dinner: Baked Flounder with Lemon and Dill
- Snack: Greek Yogurt with Fresh Peaches

Thursday

- Breakfast: Green Smoothie with Spinach, Apple, and Banana
- Lunch: Chickpea and Avocado Wrap
- Dinner: Lemon Herb Shrimp Skewers with Quinoa
- Snack: Roasted Pumpkin Seeds

Friday

- Breakfast: Oatmeal with Blueberries and Almonds
- Lunch: Mediterranean Lentil Salad
- Dinner: Grilled Salmon with Mango Salsa
- Snack: Cucumber Slices with Hummus

Saturday

- Breakfast: Mango and Pineapple Smoothie
- Lunch: Sweet Potato and Quinoa Bowl
- Dinner: Baked Snapper with Herbs and Steamed Vegetables
- Snack: Fresh Strawberries

Sunday

- Breakfast: Raspberry and Almond Butter Smoothie
- Lunch: Roasted Beet and Arugula Salad
- Dinner: Lemon Garlic Cod with Brown Rice
- Snack: Baked Apple Slices with Cinnamon

Week 9

Monday

- Breakfast: Blueberry and Oatmeal Smoothie
- Lunch: Lentil and Spinach Soup
- Dinner: Grilled Tuna Steaks with Olive Tapenade
- Snack: Pear Slices with Almond Butter

Tuesday

- Breakfast: Peach and Coconut Chia Pudding
- Lunch: Mixed Greens with Grilled Chicken and Pomegranate
- Dinner: Garlic Roasted Shrimp with Asparagus
- Snack: Carrot Sticks with Greek Yogurt Dip

Wednesday

- Breakfast: Mango and Spinach Smoothie
- Lunch: Quinoa and Black Bean Salad
- Dinner: Herb-Crusted Cod with Steamed Broccoli
- Snack: Fresh Raspberries

Thursday

- Breakfast: Banana and Walnut Overnight Oats
- Lunch: Mediterranean Chickpea Salad
- Dinner: Grilled Mahi Mahi with Pineapple Salsa
- Snack: Celery Sticks with Almond Butter

Friday

- Breakfast: Berry and Almond Butter Smoothie
- Lunch: Tomato Basil Soup
- Dinner: Lemon Garlic Grilled Shrimp with Brown Rice
- Snack: Apple Slices with Peanut Butter

Saturday

- Breakfast: Peach and Flaxseed Smoothie
- Lunch: Spiced Chickpea Stew
- Dinner: Grilled Halibut with Vegetable Medley
- Snack: Fresh Pineapple Slices

Sunday

- Breakfast: Mixed Berry Oatmeal
- Lunch: Spinach and Avocado Salad
- Dinner: Baked Salmon with Lemon and Dill
- Snack: Greek Yogurt with Honey and Walnuts

Week 10

Monday
- Breakfast: Strawberry Banana Smoothie
- Lunch: Butternut Squash Soup with Pumpkin Seeds
- Dinner: Lemon Herb Grilled Chicken with Steamed Vegetables
- Snack: Fresh Orange Slices

Tuesday
- Breakfast: Raspberry and Chia Seed Pudding
- Lunch: Quinoa and Vegetable Salad
- Dinner: Baked Cod with Lemon and Herbs
- Snack: Greek Yogurt with Fresh Berries

Wednesday
- Breakfast: Blueberry and Spinach Smoothie
- Lunch: Chickpea and Avocado Salad
- Dinner: Grilled Salmon with Asparagus
- Snack: Apple Slices with Almond Butter

Thursday
- Breakfast: Mango and Coconut Smoothie
- Lunch: Lentil and Vegetable Stew
- Dinner: Garlic Shrimp with Quinoa Pilaf
- Snack: Carrot Sticks with Hummus

Friday
- Breakfast: Peach and Almond Smoothie
- Lunch: Spinach and Strawberry Salad
- Dinner: Herb-Crusted Tilapia with Roasted Brussels Sprouts
- Snack: Celery Sticks with Greek Yogurt Dip

Saturday
- Breakfast: Berry and Flaxseed Oatmeal
- Lunch: Sweet Potato and Black Bean Chili
- Dinner: Lemon Dill Baked Haddock with Green Beans
- Snack: Fresh Raspberries

Sunday
- Breakfast: Pineapple and Spinach Smoothie
- Lunch: Roasted Beet and Goat Cheese Salad
- Dinner: Baked Sole with Lemon Butter
- Snack: Mixed Berry Salad

Weekly Meal planner+ Journal

	BREAKFAST	LUNCH	DINNER	SNACKS
MON				
TUE				
WED				
THU				
FRI				
SAT				
SUN				

Describe your current eating habits. How many meals and snacks do you usually have each day?

Weekly Meal planner+ Journal

	BREAKFAST	LUNCH	DINNER	SNACKS
MON				
TUE				
WED				
THU				
FRI				
SAT				
SUN				

What are your main goals for starting the multiple myeloma diet? How do you hope it will improve your health?

Weekly Meal planner+ Journal

	BREAKFAST	LUNCH	DINNER	SNACKS
MON				
TUE				
WED				
THU				
FRI				
SAT				
SUN				

What do you know about the nutritional needs specific to multiple myeloma patients? Are there any areas you need more information about?

....

....

....

....

....

....

Weekly Meal planner+ Journal

	BREAKFAST	LUNCH	DINNER	SNACKS
MON				
TUE				
WED				
THU				
FRI				
SAT				
SUN				

What challenges do you anticipate facing while transitioning to the multiple myeloma diet? How can you prepare for these challenges?

Weekly Meal planner+ Journal

	BREAKFAST	LUNCH	DINNER	SNACKS
MON				
TUE				
WED				
THU				
FRI				
SAT				
SUN				

Who can you rely on for support as you start this new diet? How can they help you stay motivated and on track?

....

....

....

....

....

....

Weekly Meal planner+ Journal

	BREAKFAST	LUNCH	DINNER	SNACKS
MON				
TUE				
WED				
THU				
FRI				
SAT				
SUN				

How comfortable are you with cooking and meal preparation? What new skills or recipes would you like to learn to support your diet?

Weekly Meal planner+ Journal

	BREAKFAST	LUNCH	DINNER	SNACKS
MON				
TUE				
WED				
THU				
FRI				
SAT				
SUN				

What strategies can you use when grocery shopping to ensure you buy foods that fit within the multiple myeloma diet guidelines?

Weekly Meal planner+ Journal

	BREAKFAST	LUNCH	DINNER	SNACKS
MON				
TUE				
WED				
THU				
FRI				
SAT				
SUN				

How will you handle eating out at restaurants or social events while following the multiple myeloma diet? What strategies can you use to make healthy choices?

Weekly Meal planner+ Journal

	BREAKFAST	LUNCH	DINNER	SNACKS
MON				
TUE				
WED				
THU				
FRI				
SAT				
SUN				

Think of a favorite recipe that doesn't fit the multiple myeloma diet. How can you modify it to make it healthier and compliant with your dietary needs?

Weekly Meal planner+ Journal

	BREAKFAST	LUNCH	DINNER	SNACKS
MON				
TUE				
WED				
THU				
FRI				
SAT				
SUN				

What positive changes have you already noticed or do you hope to notice by following the multiple myeloma diet? How can you celebrate and build on these successes?

Scan the QR code below to get a surprise bonus